The 30 MINUTE DIABETES Cookbook

Eat to beat diabetes with 100 easy low-carb recipes

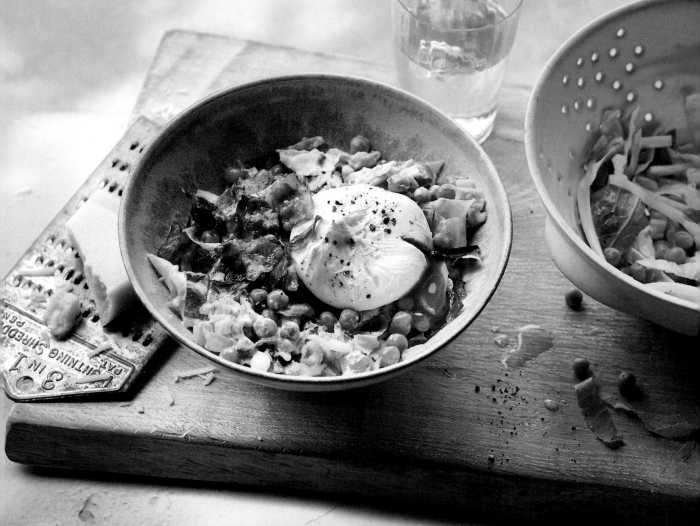

KATIE & GIANCARLO CALDESI

with Jenny Phillips

An Hachette UK Company
www.hachette.co.uk

First published in Great Britain in 2021
by Kyle Books, an imprint of Octopus Publishing Group Limited
Carmelite House
50 Victoria Embankment
London EC4Y 0DZ
www.kylebooks.co.uk

ISBN: 978 085783 918 3

Distributed in the US by Hachette Book Group, 1290 Avenue of the Americas,
4th and 5th Floors, New York, NY 10104

Distributed in Canada by Canadian Manda Group, 664 Annette St., Toronto, Ontario,
Canada M6S 2C8

Publisher: **Joanna Copestick**
Project editor: **Vicky Orchard**
Editorial assistant: **Jenny Dye**
Design: **Tina Smith Hobson**
Photography: **Maja Smend**
Food styling: **Amy Stephenson**
Props styling: **Nicole Theodorou**
Production: **Emily Noto**

A Cataloguing in Publication record for this title is available from the British Library

Printed and bound in China

10 9 8 7 6 5 4 3 2 1

Note: The information in this book is only part of how any particular person may decide which diet or indeed lifestyle is the best for them. If you are on prescribed medication or suffer from a significant medical condition, we strongly advise you to consult your own doctor before making changes. For example, improvements in lifestyle and weight loss may also significantly improve your blood pressure or diabetes control, requiring a reduction in medication. The science part of this book is written from the viewpoint of people with type 2 diabetes or those wishing to lose weight. The recipes may also be suitable for people with type 1 diabetes provided, of course, that you consult your doctor as advised above. If you are on prescribed medication, it is recommended that you check your plans with your doctor. Type 2 diabetics using insulin may well need advice about a reduction in insulin dosage to avoid the risk of a hypo.

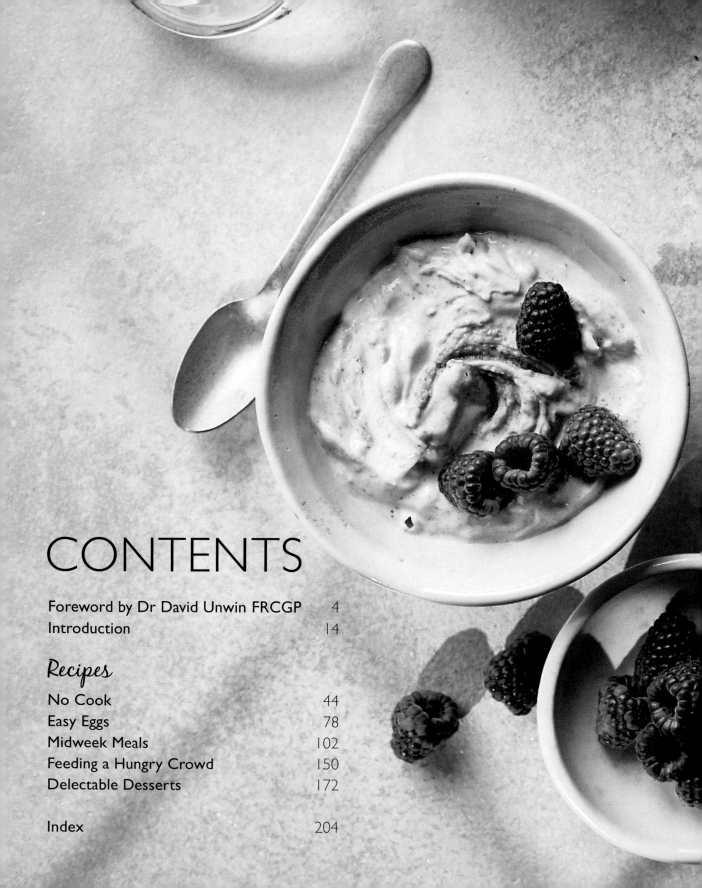

CONTENTS

FOREWORD
by Dr David Unwin

Welcome to our third low-carb cookbook. In *The Diabetes Weight-loss Cookbook* and *The Reverse Your Diabetes Cookbook*, we described how London chef Giancarlo used a low-carb diet to put his type 2 diabetes into drug-free remission with recipes devised by his cookery writer wife Katie. Since then "cutting the carbs" or "going keto" has gained yet more worldwide traction, helping people to lose weight and improve diabetic control and blood pressure while enjoying delicious food. A recent major report by the American Diabetes Association found that reducing overall carbohydrate intake for type 2 diabetics demonstrated the most evidence for improving diabetic control. This makes sense because diabetes is largely about sugar and most carbohydrates digest down into sugar. This new book shows how to reduce the carbs in your diet and improve your health by eating wonderful food – all prepared in less than 30 minutes.

I have cared for the same population of around 9,000 people as a family doctor since 1986. In that time, I have seen the effects of two terrible epidemics: obesity and type 2 diabetes. In 1986 we had 57 patients with diabetes, now there are 530. A nine-fold increase! Until 2012, I prescribed ever-increasing amounts of drugs for diabetes, but this didn't make people well. Then, one day I met someone with type 2 diabetes who, like Giancarlo, had put his diabetes into remission. In fact, he had come off all his medication and had normal blood sugar. If this miracle was possible for one person, why not for others?

As I sit at my desk today, eight years later, 82 of my patients have achieved drug-free remission from type 2 diabetes. That's 49 per cent of all those who have tried a low-carb approach, nearly one in two! On top of this, 302 people have lost an average of 10kg (22lb) in weight with improvements in their blood pressure, liver function and lipid profiles (cholesterol). Against all national trends, our practice is using fewer drugs for diabetes, saving approximately £50,000 a year. Some of the credit goes to my wife Jen, a consultant clinical psychologist, who added her skills in behaviour change and motivation, and she shares her tips with you on pages 40–43. In 2015, we teamed up with Diabetes. co.uk and helped write an online low-carb diet programme that has been downloaded by more than 440,000 people around the world. This book is about sharing all we have learned about how food can be the best medicine, and tasty into the bargain!

What is the connection between FOOD, OBESITY & DIABETES?

Over the years, I have looked after hundreds of diabetics and seen first-hand the damage diabetes can do. Until 2012, despite noticing the tsunami of extra cases, I never stopped to ask why it was happening. I noticed that people were getting much heavier and suspected that this was because they were eating more. I would now go so far as to say that 98 per cent of all cases of type 2 diabetes are caused by what we eat. Just 2 per cent are due to other factors like stress or prescribed medication. Hidden in this is my first message of hope: *you have the power to change your health as you are in control of what you eat.*

> "I would go so far as to say that 98 per cent of all cases of type 2 diabetes are caused by what we eat"

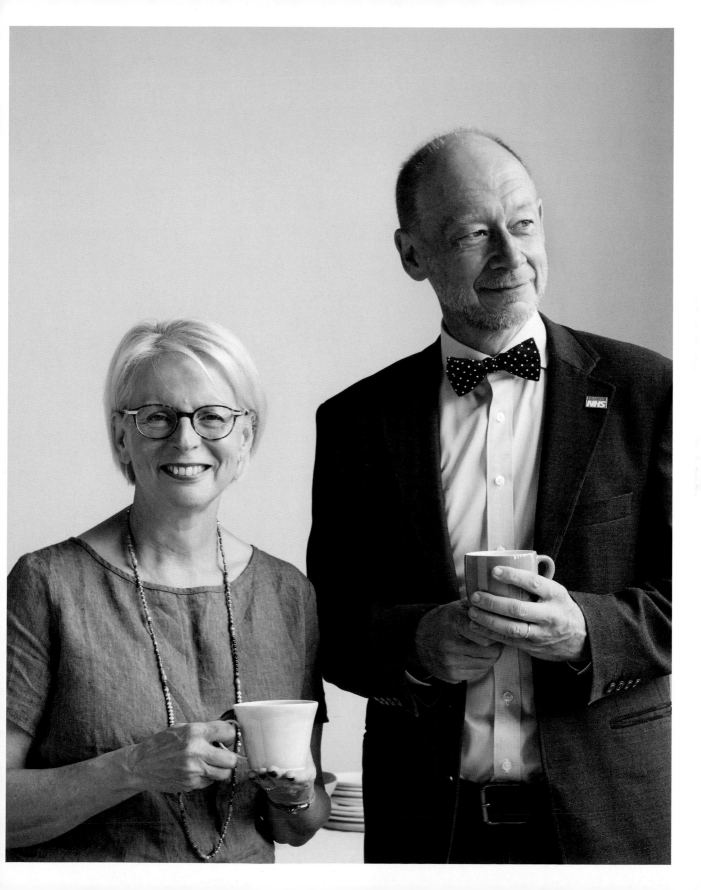

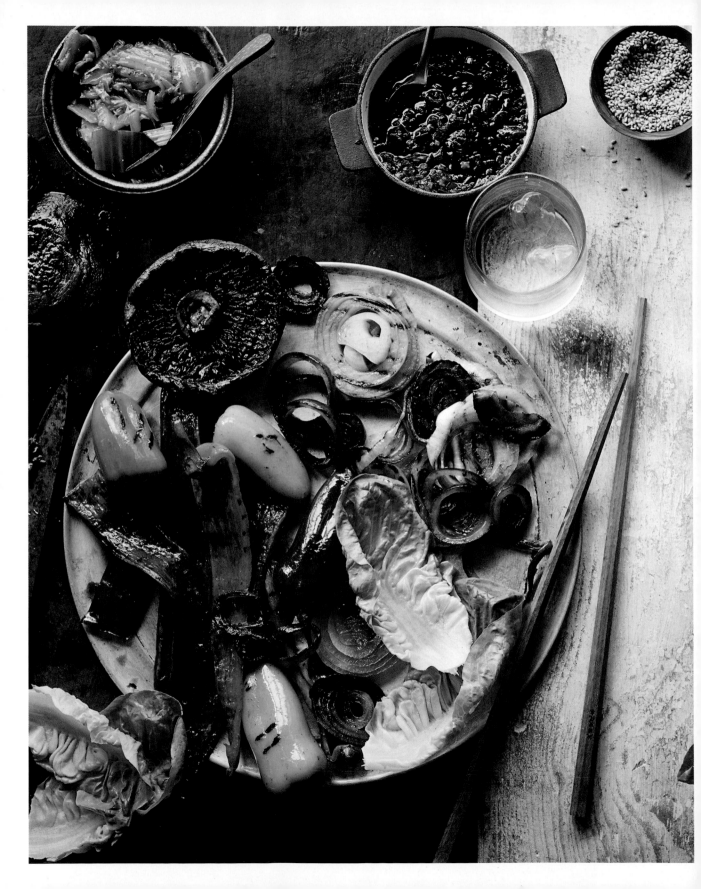

How can FOOD CAUSE DIABETES?

Let's start by explaining what diabetes is. Our bodies respond to a sugary or starchy meal by producing the hormone insulin from the pancreas or pancreatic gland. Insulin clears high blood sugar by pushing it out of the blood into muscle cells for energy. Insulin also pushes any excess sugar into belly fat and the liver, where it is converted to a fat called triglyceride. This builds up over time, causing central obesity (a big belly) and fatty liver disease. So dietary sugar becomes fat, and insulin can be seen as "fat fertilizer".

Essentially type 2 diabetics have a problem dealing with sugar (glucose) and starch (which breaks down into glucose) as either their insulin does not work properly, or they don't produce enough of it. So, glucose builds up in the bloodstream. These higher-than-normal blood sugars are a sign of diabetes and may, over time, damage small and large blood vessels in vital organs such as the eyes or kidneys. But here is my second message of hope: *if you eat less glucose, your blood sugar will be lower, and you will have better diabetic control.*

Fatty liver disease now affects 20 per cent of adults in the developed world and is becoming a third epidemic. It reduces the effectiveness of insulin (resulting in insulin resistance) and in some people sugar-derived fat also builds up in the pancreas itself, interfering with its vital role and helping to shut off the supply of insulin. Here is my third message of hope: *restricting carbohydrate-rich foods that break down into glucose by eating low carb can reverse all these fatty changes and improve pancreatic function and insulin sensitivity.*

"Rather like the new hybrid cars we have a dual-fuel engine & can burn either glucose or fat for energy"

If my DIET HAS LESS SUGAR IN IT, where will I GET MY ENERGY FROM?

The good news is that rather like the new hybrid cars we have a dual-fuel engine and can burn either glucose or fat for energy. Fat is actually a more concentrated energy source than sugar, providing 9 calories per gram compared to 4. So, why is an obese person still hungry? My average patient with type 2 diabetes weighs 100kg (nearly 16 stone) and despite having more than a month's supply of energy on board their body as fat, they are hungry for every meal and snack. Again, this is due to insulin. Because of its imperative to reduce blood sugar levels, when you eat a high-carb diet, insulin blocks your ability to burn fat, preferring sugar for fuel. This is why when I ate biscuits all day I was continually hungry, despite the fat stored in my "middle-aged spread". As I reduced the carbs in my diet, I was able to become a fat burner, burning both the fat stored in my belly and from my food.

For so many of my patients, a low-carb diet has resulted in less hunger as they start burning their own body fat. This helps to explain the keto diet. A low-carb diet contains less than 130g (4½oz) carbs a day, but if this is cut further to 50g (1¾oz) or even 30g (1oz) as on the keto diet, then nearly all your energy is coming from fat. To burn fat, your liver first has to convert it into ketones, which are then transported round the body and used as a good source of energy. You are in a state of nutritional ketosis (NOT to be confused with diabetic ketoacidosis, a dangerous and very different state sometimes found in people who cannot produce enough insulin). Intriguingly, published clinical trials demonstrate that increasing ketone availability to the brain via nutritional ketosis has a beneficial effect on cases of mild to moderate dementia.

How a LOW-CARB DIET can IMPROVE HEALTH

In the early days I worried that advising my patients to enjoy butter, eggs, meat and full-fat dairy might have some adverse effects, so I measured all the factors I could think of related to both metabolic and heart health: weight; waist circumference; total cholesterol and other lipids like HDL-cholesterol and particularly serum triglyceride; liver function (I used a blood test for the enzyme GGT for this) and blood pressure. I was astonished (and relieved) to find significant improvements in all of these areas. Thinking about insulin as a "fat fertilizer", pushing glucose into cells where it is converted into fat, then you may not be as surprised. This process leads to more belly fat and increases a particular fat called triglyceride in the liver – eventually interfering with the healthy function of the liver itself, affecting the production of blood lipids. An important meta-analysis (very large study) concluded, "Large randomized controlled trials of at least 6 months duration with carbohydrate restriction appear superior in improving lipid markers when compared with low-fat diets." In layman's terms, they found improved cholesterol in people on a low-carb diet.

But what about the improvements in blood pressure? To date, I have seen improvements in blood pressure for 196 low-carb patients as their average blood pressure reduced from 143/84mmHg to 130/77mmHg, and this is despite them coming off 20 per cent of their drugs for blood pressure!

It seems, at least in part, that high blood pressure is due to yet another function of insulin and its action on salt. We have known since 1997 that insulin causes people with diabetes to retain salt. So, a high-carb, high-insulin state causes them to retain more salt and therefore more fluid. This increases blood pressure. When they start eating low carb, many of my patients notice they are passing far more urine than normal as salt and fluid are lost. Sometimes this helps swollen ankles and abdominal bloating. One patient lost 5kg (11lb) of water-weight in just a week. It is possible we are blaming salt for what the sugar did! This also explains why we find many people actually need more salt when they start a low-carb diet.

SUGAR with your SUGAR, with your SUGAR

Type 2 diabetics have a problem dealing with a particular sugar – glucose. Glucose isn't just found in obviously sugary foods such as fruit juice or cakes but is also produced when the body breaks down starchy foods, such as rice, pasta, breakfast cereals and bread. In fact, starch is made up of glucose molecules "holding hands" and so digestion breaks it back down into surprising amounts of glucose. For example, a small bowl of cornflakes or two slices of white bread will probably affect your blood glucose in exactly the same way as 8 teaspoons of table sugar. Put like that, these are not great dietary choices for diabetics or for anyone wanting to lose weight. A breakfast of cereal, toast and fruit juice is in effect just "sugar with your sugar, with your sugar", making achieving normal blood glucose for type 2 diabetics unlikely without using drugs. By comparison a three-egg cheese omelette is the equivalent to less than 1 teaspoon of sugar.

Nutritionist Jenny Philips explains more on pages 24–34 but eating low carb essentially means cutting down on sugary and starchy foods while focusing on eating protein, good-quality fats and green vegetables instead. It's been seven years since my wife Jen and I first started offering a low-carb approach to my patients with type 2 diabetes, during which time we have developed our teaspoon of sugar graphics to rework the glycaemic load of various foods in terms of table sugar. We use these to help people make better food choices and overleaf are some we have developed recently to show you how eating different foods can affect your blood sugar.

> "Glucose isn't just found in obviously sugary foods but is also produced when the body breaks down starchy foods"

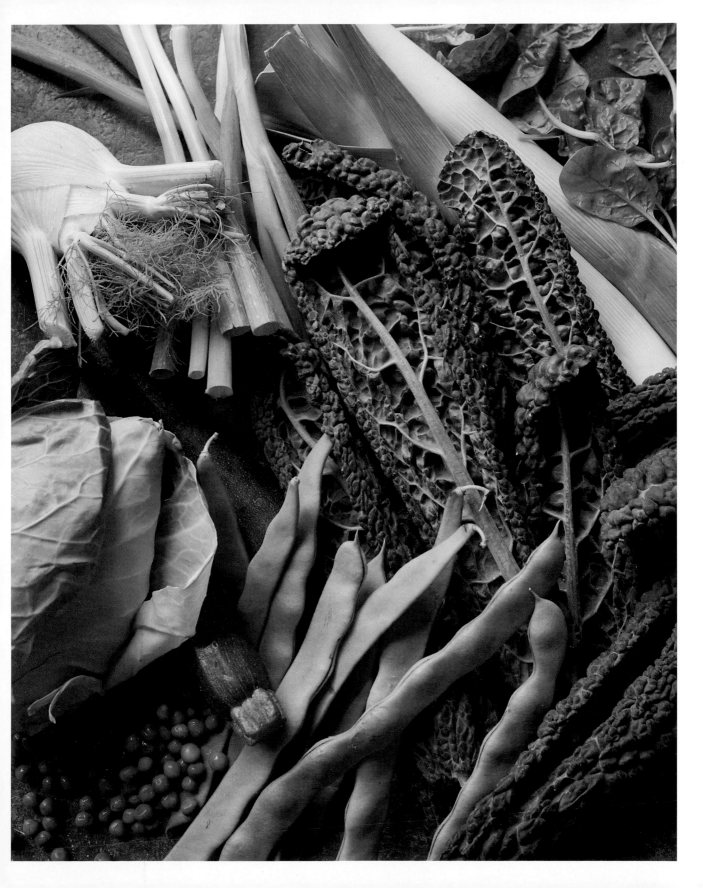

WHITE, BROWN *or* GREEN *foods?*

For years I advised my patients to switch from white bread and rice to brown alternatives as I thought these "brown carbs" were far superior to the white versions, being full of fibre and vitamins. When the patients' diabetic control was poor, I shrugged and started them on medication – completely missing the potential that these wholegrain foods have to digest down into glucose. Now I advise patients to "turn the white foods green". This means substituting carby white foods like bread, potatoes or rice with green veg like buttered broccoli or a stir-fry. The table below shows how going green rather than brown brings extra advantages in terms of reducing your sugar load.

In fact, eating green veg, meat, fish or eggs as part of a low-carb diet may be even better as not only do these

> "The longer fruit spends in the sun, the riper it becomes and the more sugar it contains"

foods all have a generally lower glycaemic load, but they are also nutritionally dense, which means they are full of vitamins, minerals, essential fatty acids and amino acids (see page 31).

White, brown or green foods?

Food	Glycaemic load (g/serve)	Serving size	How does each food affect blood glucose compared with one 4g teaspoon of table sugar?	
White rice	26	150g	9.6	～～～～～～～～～
Brown rice	20	150g	7.3	～～～～～～～
White bread	22	60g	8	～～～～～～～
Brown bread	16.2	60g	6	～～～～～
Spaghetti (white)	18	180g	6.6	～～～～～～
Spaghetti (brown)	17	180g	6.2	～～～～～～
Broccoli	0.3	250g	0.1	← Also salad leaves, courgette...

The brown bread and spaghetti are wholemeal. Rice and spaghetti boiled. 60g bread in two slices.
D Unwin *et al.*, 'It is the glycaemic response to, not the carbohydrate content of food that matters in diabetes and obesity: The glycaemic index revistited', *Journal of Insulin Resistance* 2016; 1(1), a8

FRUIT: *variably sugary*

In recent years we have been encouraged to eat our "five a day" of fruit and vegetables. Many people prefer the sweetness of fruit, so choose this over green veg. It is common for me to come across patients worried about their diabetes and weight who still believe that large amounts of fruit are healthy and that more is better. The very thing that attracts us to fruit is its sweetness, but how sugary different fruits are varies a lot. To understand this, it helps to remember that the longer fruit spends in the sun, the riper it becomes and the more sugar it contains. This means that in general tropical fruits like bananas, oranges or pineapples contain a lot more sugar than a Scottish raspberry. In general, all berries are the least sugary choice. Dried fruit like raisins are the most sugary and other fruit comes in between as shown in the table below.

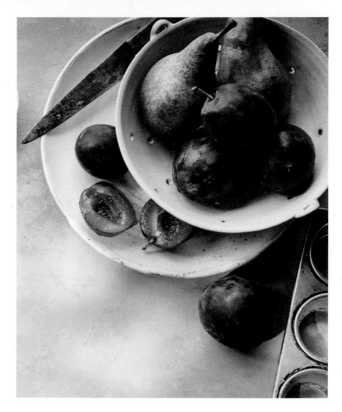

How fruit affects blood glucose

Type of fruit	GI from scientific literature	Serve size	Glycaemic load (g/serve)	How does 120g of each fruit affect blood glucose compared with one 4g teaspoon of table sugar?	
Banana	26	120g	16	5.9	〰〰〰〰〰〰
Grapes, black	20	120g	11	4.0	〰〰〰〰
Apple, golden delicious	22	120g	6	2.2	〰〰
Watermelon, fresh	16.2	120g	5	1.8	〰〰
Nectarines, fresh	18	120g	4	1.5	〰〰
Apricots, fresh	17	120g	3	1.1	〰
Strawberries, fresh	0.3	120g	3.8	1.4	〰

The glycaemic index helps predict how these fruits might affect blood glucose, important information if you have type 2 diabetes.
As per calculations to be found in D Unwin et al., 'It is the glycaemic response to, not the carbohydrate content of food that matters in diabetes and obesity: The glycaemic index revistited', *Journal of Insulin Resistance* 2016; 1(1), a8 @lowcarbGP

EGGS: a CHEAP SOURCE of LOW-CARB NUTRIENTS

Due to worries about cholesterol, for years I advised my patients to cut back on eggs in their diet or try (the rather tragic) yolkless omelettes. I remember advising no more than two whole eggs a week as a treat! However, when I retested their cholesterol levels, I was so often disappointed that their sacrifice did not seem to be rewarded in their blood test results. Then in 2013 I saw a study in the journal *Metabolism* where they gave three eggs a day to people with type 2 diabetes and found significant improvements in cholesterol and other important blood fats. On top of this there was an improvement in diabetes control. So, goodbye horrid yolkless omelettes!

Can I eat a LOW-CARB DIET if I'm on prescribed MEDICATION?

This book is not here to replace the individual advice given by your GP or practice nurse which is based on your own specific case and medical history. In general, if you are on prescribed medication, please check any major dietary changes with your prescribing doctor. This is particularly relevant for the following:

Firstly, drugs prescribed for hypertension (high blood pressure). It is possible that your blood pressure could improve so much as to make these drugs unnecessary, or even bring about a postural drop in blood pressure that could make you feel dizzy. So, bear this in mind and monitor blood pressure if you're on BP-lowering meds.

Secondly, for those taking drugs for diabetes, is there a risk of lowering the blood sugar too much? This is an obvious risk for those using insulin, but other drugs also

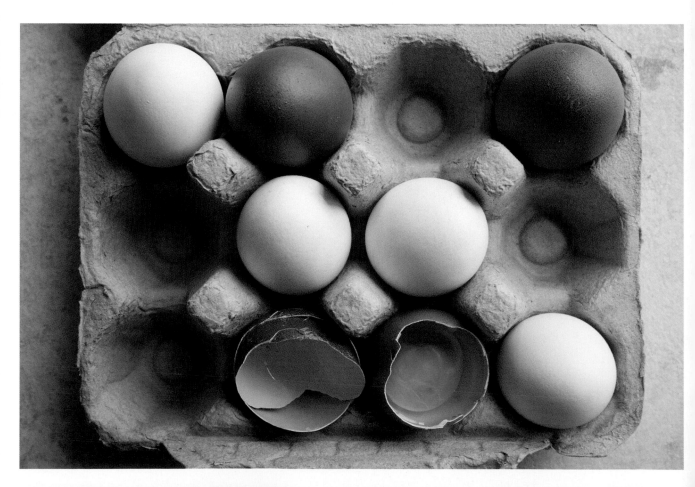

have this potential problem (although not metformin, which is a very commonly used drug for type 2 diabetes and safe with a low-carb diet). There is a different risk in the form of diabetic ketoacidosis for those on the new SGLT2 inhibitor drugs (such as canagliflozin and dapagliflozin). In my opinion, it is not safe to be both low carb and on SGLT2i drugs.

A word about CARB CREEP

For many of my patients, eating low carb is a lifestyle, rather than a diet that they are on for just a few weeks. My longest low-carb patient started the approach years before me in 2003, and he is still in drug-free type 2 diabetes remission 17 years later! But do bear in mind that some people make a great start only to find their weight increasing and blood sugars rising a few months later, often after Christmas or a holiday. At this point, sometimes doctors feel that their change in diet has failed and start medication. But so often there's no need to despair. In fact, for most people the diet hasn't "failed", but they have just started allowing carbs to creep back into their diet and so aren't really low carb any more. I ask these patients about the possibility of "carb creep" and whether they want to start drugs or revisit their diet. Almost without exception they go back to eating low carb, but with lessons learned that mean they do it even better. As my wife Jen explains on pages 40–43, "going low carb is simple, but it's not always easy".

In every clinic I'm seeing people who have transformed their health and their lives by cutting out sugar and starchy carbs. I really hope this book helps you find a way to a healthier future. My patients often tell me it's a permanent lifestyle not a diet and I wholeheartedly agree!

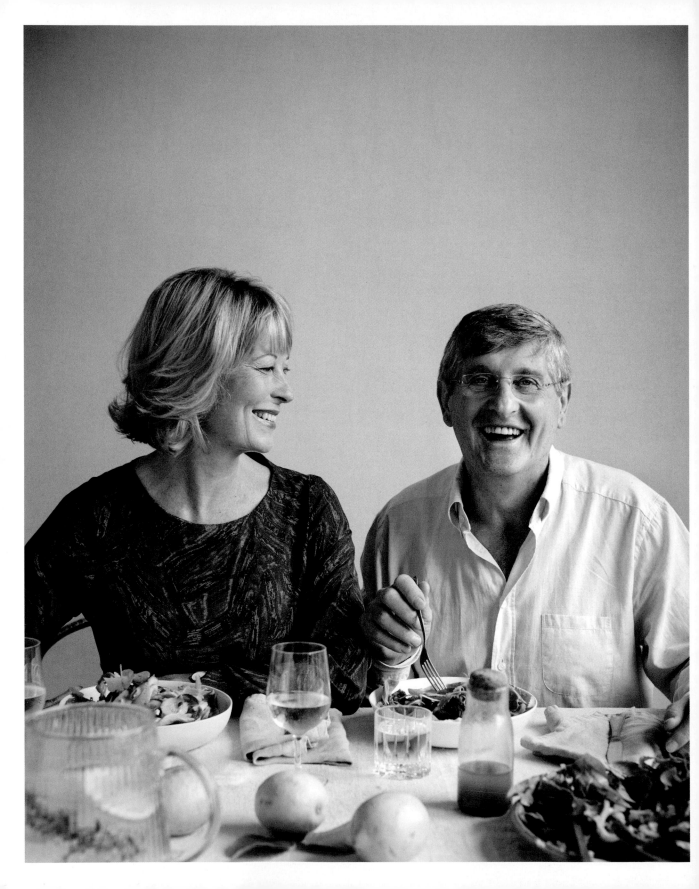

KATIE & GIANCARLO
making the change

We recently bought a new vacuum cleaner. It was a family decision; one son researched the options, we all discussed it, made our choice and after a couple of days it arrived. It has changed the way we clean, the way our house looks and we are all delighted. The old one was heavy, bulky, got stuck on corners and mostly made us grumpy to use it, so we rarely did. Why did it take us 15 years to do this?

Giancarlo and I were discussing this simple decision and change and likened it to him having type 2 diabetes for ten years. The old heavy, grumpy Giancarlo who couldn't move around easily compared to the new, lighter one who makes us all happy. It might sound amusing and flippant to compare my husband to a vacuum cleaner, but there is a simple message here: *don't put up with things if they are not right*. Giancarlo became used to his body not working properly and thought it was just "being middle-aged". Until we did our own research and talked to other people, he didn't know he could have a sparkling, all-singing, all-dancing version of himself by committing to changing what he ate.

It has been eight years since we started eating a low-carb diet 95 per cent of the time. Since we run Italian restaurants and love our food, we will always enjoy the occasional bowl of fresh pasta or a slice of pizza straight from the oven, but it is a rarity not a daily occurrence. We always make sure there are low-carb options for our customers and ourselves so that everyone can avoid temptation easily.

Living a low-carb life keeps Giancarlo's type 2 diabetes in remission. From an HBa1C of 79 mmol/mol in 2013, he is now a steady 39 mmol/mol having had his last test in October 2020. I suffered from irritable bowel syndrome (IBS) and was overweight. I have lost a stone and kept it off and the IBS has gone. Our sons are lean, we are all fitter and healthier despite being older and all of us have noticed our skin is better. It is exciting, moving and heart-warming to hear from others who have gone low carb and are in remission from type 2 diabetes. Simply by making better food choices we have carved healthier lives for ourselves without the need for medication. If we can do it with all the temptations around us, then so can you.

Giancarlo says that when you first cut out sugar and carbs it might seem like a struggle but remind yourself every day you manage it that you have achieved your goal and feel good about that. You will soon reap the health benefits and the cravings will lessen. Giancarlo does enjoy the occasional sweet treat but if he overdoes it, then his old symptoms return. He knows he is only in remission from type 2 diabetes because of living a low-carb lifestyle and is determined to stay well for a bright and happy future.

> "If we can do it with all the temptations around us, then so can you"

How did we create THESE RECIPES?

I asked nutritionist Jenny Phillips to help put together a few recipe guidelines when I started writing this book. It helped keep me on track and I am sure it will be useful for you too.

1 **Exclude starchy carbohydrate** foods and sugars, both of which cause a rapid rise in blood sugar. These include bread, pasta, potato, noodles (unless low carb), rice, wheat flour used in baking, such as traditional pizza bases, oats, couscous and other grains, and sugar (see point 9 for how to add a little natural sweetness when required).

2 **Substitute starchy foods** for alternatives based on nuts, seeds, vegetables and a limited use of gram (chickpea) flour where required for authenticity.

3 **Protein is a very important part** of every meal; it is used by the body for growth and repair. Vegetarians need to carefully ensure they are consuming adequate protein from pulses, cheese, nuts, seeds and eggs. Flexitarians have the advantage of meat and fish, which are incredibly nutritious and good sources of vitamin B12, iron and essential fats. Enjoy red meat, including good-quality (ie high- meat-content) sausages and bacon.

4 **Here's the good news** – you can include generous amounts of good fats within the dishes. These are essential for metabolism and help you to feel fuller for longer. Oily fish, such as salmon, mackerel, sardines and anchovies, contain omega 3, which helps to reduce inflammation and keep your brain healthy. Use extra virgin olive oil in salad dressings and for light frying. Butter, ghee, dripping and coconut oil are all tasty saturated fats which are safe to heat in roasting and frying. Avoid margarines and vegetable oils which oxidize when heated. Also avoid low-fat products which tend to include sugars and sweeteners to improve their flavour. Full-fat Greek yogurt is a good choice.

5 **Enjoy lots of vegetables** with every meal. Include generous amounts of non-starchy and salad vegetables to ensure you feel full.

6 **Sauces are a great way** to increase your calorie intake to compensate for the absence of starchy carbs and grains and to enhance the flavour and enjoyment of meals.

7 **Starchy vegetables are a good replacement** for grains and potatoes – these tend to be vegetables that grow underground such as celeriac, turnips, swede, carrots, pumpkin, butternut squash and beetroot. Exclude potatoes, parsnips and sweet potatoes because of their higher carb content.

Counting the carbs in starchy veg
(g carbs per 100g)

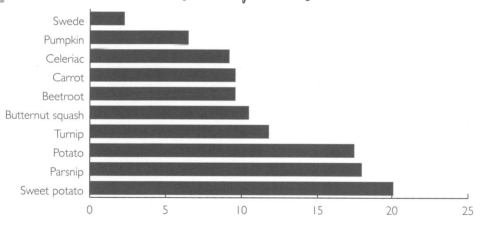

8 **When it comes to fruit,** berries are a good choice as they are naturally low in sugar. Your choice of other fruit depends on where you are on the CarbScale (see page 29). Modest quantities of fruit within a salad or alongside a main course add flavour and interest. Go slow on high-sugar tropical fruits such as mango, pineapple and banana.

9 **Where a dish requires a little sweetness,** use a small amount of dried fruit (dates or apricots) or a little honey. Per serving this will have a negligible effect on your blood sugar.

10 **Enjoy some low-carb celebration** or dessert dishes. Double cream is allowed!

How to USE THIS BOOK

The chapters are not separated into breakfast, lunch and dinner as most of us no longer eat in such a traditional way. Depending on what we've got on, we can now easily flex our mealtimes and frequency of eating. We don't snack between meals or graze our way through the day.

Often, Giancarlo and I skip breakfast and enjoy a substantial brunch late morning which keeps us powered for the day. Alternatively, we eat eggs for breakfast or just have a coffee with cream and enjoy a light lunch. We try to enjoy a family mealtime in the evening so that we can all catch up on our day. Feel free to mix and match these recipes to fit in with your schedule and commitments.

Calculating CARBS

I have given the nutritional analysis at the bottom of each recipe. As ingredients vary so much this is only a guide, but it will help you see the nutritional value of the meals in respect of carbs, protein and fats. You can use various software to calculate carbs (and there are discrepancies between them) or the Carbs and Cals app or book. Alternatively I find it a good idea to look at what you are eating and imagine it as a pile of ingredients or read the label – if it was originally low-carb ingredients such as a few almonds, a vegetable, an egg, meat or fish with a little flavouring then go ahead and eat it. If it was a pile of wheat flour or rice originally, or contains poor-quality fat, sugar and various additives, then it will be high in carbs so don't.

In essence keep carbs fairly low (depending on where you are on the CarbScale – see page 29), enjoy good-quality protein (see page 31 for recommended daily intake) and be generous with good fats. Your goal is to switch your metabolism from storing fat to burning fat as an efficient energy source.

GET ahead

Always read the recipe all the way through first. Since every dish is cooked in 30 minutes or less, get all the ingredients out in front of you so you know if anything is missing before you start cooking. I have given plenty of swaps, particularly as I wrote this book during lockdown when it was hard to find certain ingredients and to shop regularly. Popping out for basil wasn't an option when parsley would do! I learned an important lesson from Cambodian chef Susie Jones about adapting recipes according to what you have in your fridge. She showed me some Asian salads but explained rather than hunt down a rare Thai fruit or vegetable, she would think about what its job was in the dish. She used shavings of raw swede for crunch, cherries for sweetness and a lime for sourness. None of them were in the original recipe but they did the same job.

TIMINGS

Where one food can be cooking while you prepare the remaining ingredients, I have suggested that. Most of the recipes should be easy to make within 30 minutes on your own. Some of the recipes are a combination of flavours, a flurry of leaves and a quick dressing or some are simply an assembly of ingredients with no cooking at all. Others may require a little team assistance but isn't that part of the fun? You are going to cook fast; think rapid boils, microwaves and time-saving food processors. It is all about getting the food from the cupboard and fridge to the table within 30 minutes.

> "Often, Giancarlo and I skip breakfast and enjoy a substantial brunch late morning which keeps us powered for the day"

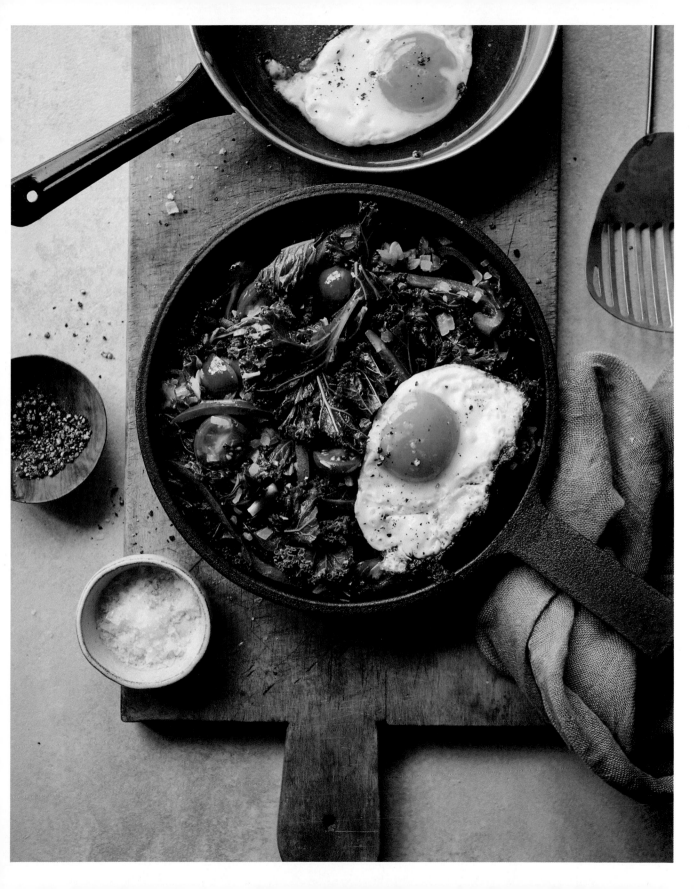

Storecupboard HEROINES

My experiences of working with women from different cultures in their home kitchens has helped me to open my mind to different ingredients. It has also introduced me to their time-saving tips and quick meals. Now with eggs permanently on hand, my essential storecupboard ingredients and my always-in-the-fridge foods, I can always rustle up a quick dish without ever resorting to ready meals.

ALWAYS-IN-THE-FRIDGE Foods

Greek yogurt

Double cream

Salted or unsalted butter made from milk from grass-fed cows – either is fine for any of the recipes

Parmesan or Grana Padano, Cheddar, cream cheese

Vegetables – cabbages, spring onions, lettuce, carrots, peppers, aubergines, cucumber, celery, cauliflower

Lemons

Harissa paste – seek out a good variety that you like made from chilli, salt and oil

Horseradish sauce

Nuts – pine nuts, walnuts, almonds, pecans and macadamia are best stored in the freezer for instant flavour and crunch

Flaxseed – golden gives a good colour to baking; keep it in the fridge to stop it becoming rancid

By the HOB

Extra virgin olive oil – I keep two types, one standard variety for cooking and one more expensive single-estate oil for drizzling over cooked foods and salads

Black pepper from a good peppermill

Fine sea salt, preferably without an anti-caking agent as I believe you get a better distribution of flavour than salt flakes which are also expensive

Eggs – I use medium in the recipes

Tomatoes – stored out of the fridge for the best flavour

Onions and garlic

"Now, I can always rustle up a quick dish without ever resorting to ready-meals"

In the CUPBOARD

Baking powder – we look for a gluten-free version

Psyllium husk (coarse not powder) – available from health food shops and online

Coconut flour – find it in larger supermarkets and health food shops

Ground almonds

Vanilla extract – preferably without sugar but that can be hard to find or expensive and I use a lot!

Canned and frozen low-carb fruit

Canned beans, lentils, chickpeas

Canned tomatoes – a good Italian brand

Canned sardines, mackerel, tuna and pilchards

Roast peppers in a jar or make your own (see box below)

Dijon, wholegrain and English mustard – for an instant low-carb kick

A range of vinegars – but actually just red wine or cider vinegar would do and a medium-priced balsamic

Coconut oil, ghee (I make my own), **dripping** (saved fat from roast meat)

Dried lentils, chickpeas, beans

Peanut butter and tahini

Tamari (gluten free) or soy sauce

Worcestershire sauce

Toasted sesame oil

Toasted sesame seeds – toast plenty and keep them in a jar for instant flavour and crunch

Spices – ground coriander, cumin and turmeric, curry powder, chaat masala powder, chilli flakes, smoked paprika, paprika, black onion (nigella) seeds, fennel seeds

HERBS

Almost every Italian household manages to grow at least two herbs; rosemary and thyme keep going in small pots on the window ledges of tiny apartments or in grand gardens throughout the year. I add flat-leaf parsley into that mix and in summer they are joined by basil and a chilli plant. Herbs are cheap and make a massive difference to the flavour and look of recipes. A scattering of chopped fresh herbs lifts the bland to the memorable.

Keep celery leaves from a bunch of celery. They can be used anywhere instead of flat-leaf parsley and basil; try them stirred into scrambled eggs or scattered over soups.

> "A scattering of chopped fresh herbs lifts the bland to the memorable"

Roast PEPPERS

While travelling and cooking in Bulgaria we used a lot of roast peppers. You can find good ones in Polish shops or make your own. Roast whole red peppers in the oven at 240°C/220°C fan/475°F/gas mark 9 for 45 minutes or until blackened. Try to do this while using the oven for another recipe. Put the cooked peppers into a bowl and cover with a large plate. Set aside for 20 minutes, then peel off the skin and discard the seeds and core. Store in the fridge for up to 4 days or in the freezer for up to 3 months.

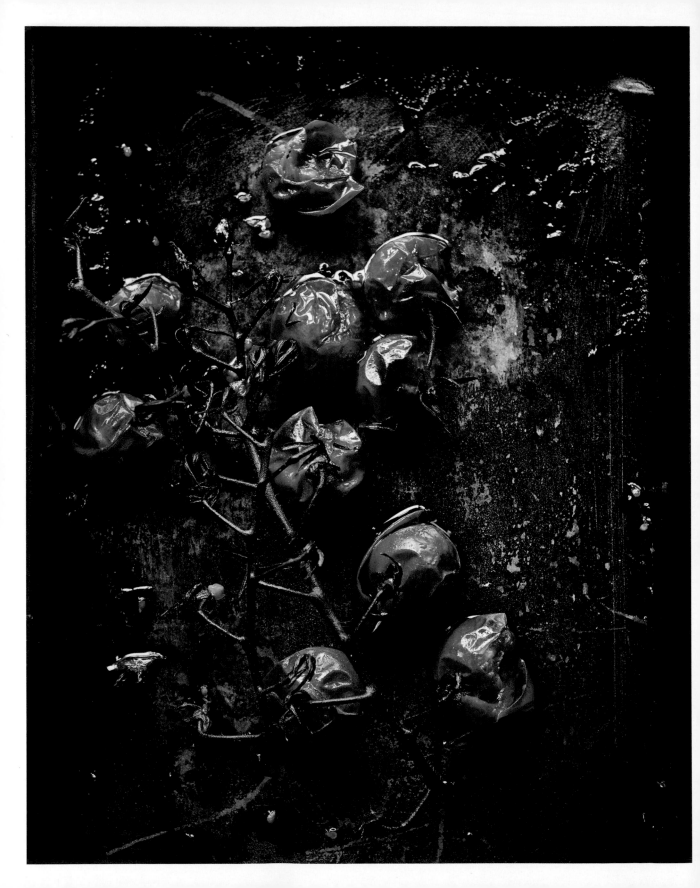

Energy-saving WAYS TO COOK

These recipes don't always start with preheating the oven. This is because, with an eye on energy efficiency, I now preheat my oven just minutes before I need it. Make a mental note of how long it takes for your oven to heat up; mine takes just 8 minutes to get to 220°C/200°C fan/425°F/gas mark 7, so there is no need for it to be on 30 minutes before I need it. You can also put food in the oven as it warms up.

Most households have a microwave and these are great for speed and using only a small amount of energy.

Cooking OVER FIRE

I have included a few recipes that can be cooked over a barbecue, but they can also be cooked under a grill inside. During lockdown, like many, we entertained outside and cooked over a fire. It is a habit that we have continued. It takes a bit of a push to make yourself go outside and light the fire, but the benefits are amazing: fresh air, being together away from screens and great-tasting food. We have done comparisons with the flavour of the indoor grill and outdoor fire and they are so different.

> "It takes a bit of a push to make yourself go outside & light the fire, but the benefits are amazing: fresh air, being together away from screens & great-tasting food"

Use the WHOLE VEGETABLE

● **When using spring onions** do use the white and green parts. Save the roots and tips for stock.

● **Use broccoli and cauliflower stalks** in the Creamy Vegetable Soup on page 107.

● **Use cauliflower leaves** to make cauliflower rice (page 124).

● **Use any cabbage leaves**, the outer leaves of sprouts as well as the tops and leaves and cauliflower leaves in the Cheesy Garlicky Kale Crisps on page 157.

● **Use beetroot leaves and foraged ground elder** (make sure you know what you are picking) instead of spinach.

We have chickens that love our vegetable peelings and other scraps, but I keep carrot, celeriac, celery and onion peelings in a bag in the freezer. When I have enough, I make a vegetable stock or add in roast bones for chicken or meat stocks. Stocks are the building blocks for so many other recipes, such as soups, casseroles, sauces and gravy, and we benefit from the nutrition, in particular the collagen from bone broths.

For a more thorough list of foods, sourcing and tips on cooking see our website **www.lowcarbtogether.com**

LOW CARB
nutritious, delicious & super-fast

Jenny Phillips, nutritionist

Eighteen years ago, I seriously transformed my diet. At just 39 years old, I was diagnosed and treated for cancer, and so began my discovery of how food can help to either hurt or heal your body.

I was lucky that my treatment was successful, and the name of the game then became "how do I stop it coming back?" Recurrence is always a worry once you've had cancer, and my risk was put at 50:50. Not odds that I liked. So, both to help my recovery, and as an insurance policy for the future, I turned to food with the aim of creating the healthiest version of me. With a degree in chemistry, I was able to delve into the science and learn how best to fuel my body. I learned a lot and was horrified that my diet, based on the so-called "Eat Well" guidelines, could be so off the mark.

One of the most powerful things I learned is that a lot of us are overfed and under-nourished. We are encouraged to "base our meals on starchy carbohydrates" like bread, pasta, cereals, rice and potatoes. Yet these are the very foods that our bodies break down quickly, sending our blood sugar levels soaring and driving an insatiable appetite which sets the scene for overeating. At the same time, such foods deliver less vitamins, minerals, essential amino acids (from protein) and healthy fats that our bodies need to function. Add to that the increased availability of hyper-palatable processed foods and it's not hard to see why our modern diets can have all sorts of negative health ramifications.

Working with the Caldesis and the Unwins, alongside my nutrition clients, has confirmed that eating low carb meals based around high-nutrient ingredients is the key to improving health and wellbeing.

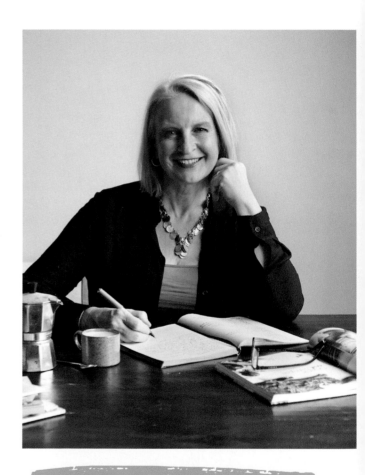

"One of the most powerful things I learned is that a lot of us are overfed & under-nourished"

METABOLIC HEALTH
what it is & why it matters

Your metabolism is the sum of all the biochemical processes that run your body; day in, day out. This includes the way that your cells produce energy from food, which powers both the unconscious processes which keep you alive (making hormones, digesting, building muscle etc) and those that you are aware of, such as movement and exercise.

You are metabolically healthy if you release the energy from digestion easily, using it in your cells to power your body. You feel well, can exercise easily and are lean, especially around your middle (weight gain around the belly is also known as central obesity). It may surprise you to know that in the US only 12 per cent of the population is metabolically healthy.

Type 2 diabetes is a metabolically unhealthy condition, where one of your fuels, glucose (from eating sugar or starchy carbs), rises in the bloodstream and can have trouble entering your cells. Excess glucose is escorted to your liver via the hormone insulin and stored either as glycogen in the muscles and liver, or as fat, which builds up around your middle. The end result is a double whammy – you gain weight around your abdomen but may feel constantly tired as your carby calories are stored as fat and not used for fuel.

Although the consequence of eating processed and refined carbohydrates for many is weight gain, the slim among us are not automatically immune. You may have heard of the acronym TOFI – Thin on the Outside, Fat on the Inside – where visceral fat builds up in the abdomen and around organs like the heart even when bodyweight is in the normal range. A build-up of this visceral fat increases your risk of type 2 diabetes and heart disease.

What is INSULIN?

This crucial hormone regulates your blood sugar levels by moving glucose from the bloodstream into your cells where it's used as fuel. When you eat too much glucose, from sugary or starchy foods, insulin levels are consistently high, and your body becomes increasingly unable to manage your glucose levels. This is known as insulin resistance and results in fat storage around your organs. High insulin levels are linked to an increased risk of many chronic diseases such as type 2 diabetes and heart disease

What is BMR?

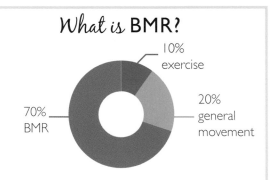

70% BMR
10% exercise
20% general movement

Basal Metabolic Rate is the amount of energy you expend while at rest. It includes the calories required to perform all life-sustaining biochemical processes. On average it is about 1,400 calories for women and 1,800 calories for men (about 70 per cent of your total energy expenditure). So, if you are reducing your calorie intake, you need to ensure that you are not negatively impacting your metabolism.

The current advice to "eat less and move more" is hard when you may already be feeling below par. Instead, you need to think like a racehorse owner or Formula 1 driver and find the best fuel to enhance your performance. (OK, we're not wanting you to turn into an Olympic athlete but feeling energized and able to enjoy daily activities is the sort of performance that can make a world of difference to your everyday life!). Good metabolic health matters because you become efficient at releasing energy from your food and feel healthier as a result. The even better news is that it can also increase your lifespan as your risk of cardiovascular disease and other complications, such as type 2 diabetes, decreases.

Low-carb SUPER FUEL

Low carb is an eating style which minimizes the consumption of high-sugar and high-carbohydrate starchy foods. This is because carbohydrates are made up of long chains of glucose molecules, which break down surprisingly quickly and increase both blood sugar and insulin levels.

To understand why this is a problem, consider the following: at any point in time you have about 1 teaspoon of sugar circulating in your bloodstream. When you eat sugar and starchy carbs, glucose is quickly released from these foods and absorbed into your blood in quantities that make it difficult for your body to deal with. For example, using Dr Unwin's sugar chart (see page 10) you can see that a portion of rice breaks down to the equivalent of 10 teaspoons of sugar! Even

"low carb puts real foods & natural ingredients centre stage"

a metabolically healthy person will find that their blood sugar will spike with starchy foods, but if you have type 2 diabetes it is harder to recover your blood sugar control. The more frequently you consume these foods, the more likely you are to increase your insulin resistance (see page 25) and this can lead to the development of prediabetes or type 2 diabetes.

But if you reduce your carbs, where do you get your energy from? When eating low carb you derive much of your energy from your second source of food-based fuel – fat. After many decades of fearing fat, this might sound strange or even alarming. However, eating low carb is incredibly safe and actually quite normal – wind the clock back 70 years or so and it is the way your grandmother would have eaten. Rather than relying on refined and processed foods, low carb puts real foods and natural ingredients centre stage. There is a double bonus to eating more foods that are naturally higher in fat, like dairy, eggs and meat. Firstly, blood glucose levels remain stable and insulin levels are reduced. Secondly, fat tends to fill you up. So, you can improve your metabolic health, lose weight if you need to and reduce your taste for sweet and starchy foods.

STARCHY CARBS are SUGAR MOLECULES "holding hands"

$CH_2 OH$ $CH_2 OH$ $CH_2 OH$

OH   OH   OH

OH   OH   OH

Know your CARBS

High-sugar foods	High-carb foods	Low-carb foods
Biscuits	Pizza	Meat
Cake	Pasta	Fish
Sweets	Bread	Eggs
Milk chocolate	Cereals containing oats	Green vegetables
Fizzy drinks	Rice	Mushrooms
Ice cream	Pastries and baked goods	Nuts and seeds
Commercial milk shakes	Crisps	Oils and fats
Fruit juices	Potatoes	Yogurt, butter, cheese and other dairy products
Dried fruit		

Your METABOLIC HEALTH

As Dr Unwin discusses on page 8, there are five factors to look at when assessing your metabolic health. These often start to improve when you switch to eating low carb.

● Blood sugars are stabilized because you're not eating foods that cause spikes.

● Your liver doesn't need to store excess glucose (from sugars and starchy carbs) as triglycerides or fats which travel in your blood.

● Therefore fat doesn't accumulate around your waist.

● Lower blood glucose means lower insulin levels, which reduces sodium retention (the storage of salt) and helps to normalize your blood pressure.

● HDL, your "good" cholesterol, improves, and this is a better predictor of your future heart attack risk than total cholesterol.

Your LOW-CARB MENU

The difference between low-carb and low-calorie diets is that eating low carb is an abundant way to enjoy your meals, which is why so many people find it is a sustainable lifestyle change which leaves them feeling energized, healthy and happy. The focus is on filling up on natural foods that keep blood sugar and insulin levels low, while delivering the fuel and nutrients – proteins, essential fats, vitamins and minerals – to power your body through the day.

"Low carb is an eating style which suits many people & can be flexed for different health goals"

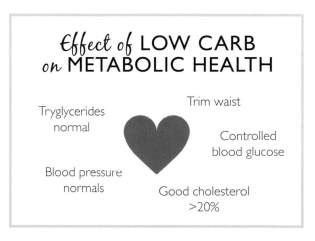

Effect of LOW CARB on METABOLIC HEALTH

Tryglycerides normal

Trim waist

Controlled blood glucose

Blood pressure normals

Good cholesterol >20%

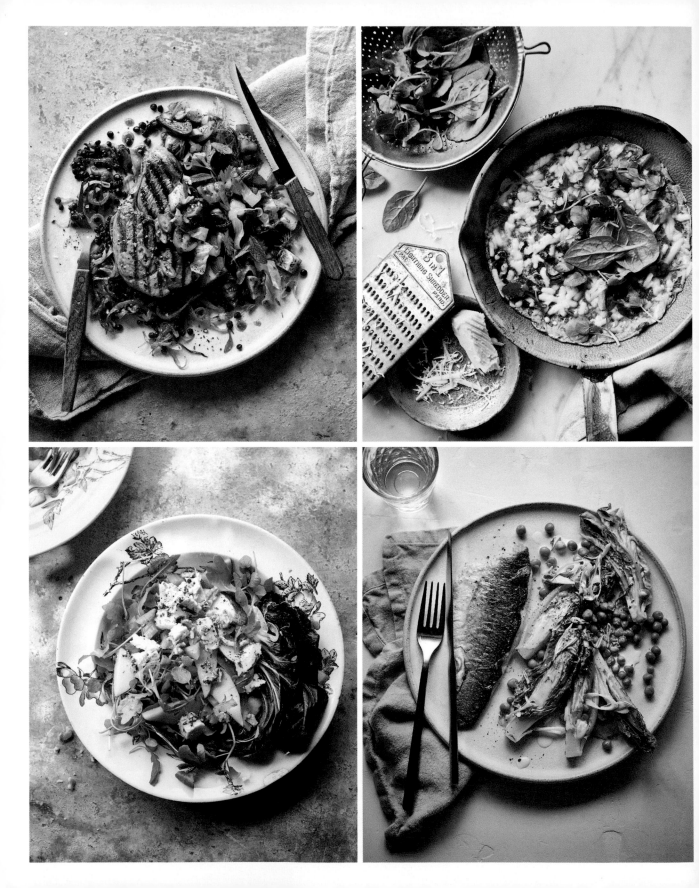

THE MACRONUTRIENTS:
carbs, protein & fats

Macronutrients are those nutrients we require in larger quantities to build strong, healthy bodies and power them with a good fuel supply. The meal plans (see page 36) are designed to help you make choices that improve your metabolic health. You will also find that each of the recipes in this book has nutritional information which lists the carbs, protein and fat per portion to help you plan your own menus.

LOW-CARB FOODS for
maintaining stable blood sugar

Carbs are energy providers, but fuelling your body with a high-carb intake can come at a price (see page 35). Concentrated sources of carbohydrates can, over time, cause wildly fluctuating blood sugar and insulin levels leading to prediabetes, type 2 diabetes and other complications like cardiovascular disease.

HOW DO FATS & CARBS
affect blood glucose levels?

This blood sugar reading, from a non-diabetic, shows clearly how low-carb meals – for breakfast and lunch – maintain steady blood glucose levels. However, eating a high-carb, healthy-looking cereal bar late in the afternoon causes a rapid spike in blood sugar.

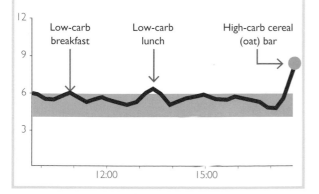

THE CARBSCALE
flexing your carb intake
to meet your needs

The good news is that low carb is an eating style which suits many people and can be flexed for different health goals. In *The Diabetes Weight-loss Cookbook* we introduced the CarbScale to show how this can work. Limit your carbohydrate intake to a daily maximum of 130g (4½oz); if you are diabetic or looking to improve your metabolic health, then you might want to reduce your intake to 50g (1¾oz) per day.

Liberal low carb
up to 130g (4½oz) carbs a day
Suitable for metabolically healthy people, this allows a more generous inclusion of starchy carbs like fruit, starchy veg and some wholegrains.

Moderate low carb
75–100g (2¾–3½oz) carbs a day
A starting point for reducing carbs, this bases meals on protein and non-starchy veg and allows some fruit and starchy veg, but not grains (which are the starchiest foods of all).

Strict low carb
50g (1¾oz) carbs a day
This is a more restricted diet and eliminates all starchy carbs – grains, most fruit and starchy veg. It is a more therapeutic diet for the experienced low carber who is looking to improve metabolic health and/or lose weight. If weight loss is not your goal, then calories are added as fat, for instance adding butter to vegetables.

The CarbScale allows families and friends to eat meals together by flexing the carb element. Once you become familiar with where the carbs are hidden, you can manage just by using the guidelines (see page 30) rather than counting carbs.

Top tips to
REDUCE CARBS

1 **Avoid sugary foods** like cakes, biscuits, or sweets. Instead make some low-carb desserts and cakes (see pages 172–203); if you are watching your weight then go easy, but these recipes won't wreak havoc with your blood sugar and insulin levels:

2 **Avoid high-carb foods** like pizza, pasta, potatoes (even sweet ones), rice, bread and cereals. Don't panic – we know that these foods may make up a significant part of your current diet. Eating good-quality protein and healthy fats alongside lots of vegetables will fill you up and help you feel that way for longer.

3 **Fill your plate with non-starchy vegetables** – as Dr Unwin often says, "turn the white food green". Vegetables add bulk, variety and flavour, and are a source of slow-release carbs that your body can handle. They are also a good source of soluble fibre, which helps healthy digestion.

4 **Enjoy root vegetables too**, which can add a comfort factor in place of starchier options like potatoes or pasta.

5 **Fruit is a naturally healthy food** provided you are metabolically healthy and depending on where you are on the CarbScale (see page 29). Berries are the lowest carb fruits, and bananas, unfortunately, are one of the highest (a small banana delivers the equivalent of 6 teaspoons of sugar!) Whole fruits are better than juiced, see below. All dried fruits are very sugary.

6 **Milk contains 5g (⅛oz) carbs** per 100ml (3½fl oz), so try to limit it you are really reducing your carb intake – enjoy an Americano rather than a cappuccino or use cream in your coffee instead.

7 **Alcohol can be a surprising hidden source of carbs** – the worst offenders are beer, lager and cider. Wine, champagne or spirits are lower carb options. Try to keep within the drinking guidelines, which recommend 14 units of alcohol per week. This is equivalent to four 250ml (9fl oz) glasses of wine, or seven 50ml (2fl oz) shots of a spirit such as gin. Be careful with mixers – low-calorie options are a better choice to avoid spiking blood sugars.

8 **Fruit juices and fizzy drinks** are a serious source of sugar, containing up to 9 teaspoons of sugar per glass (250ml/9fl oz). Drink still or sparkling water, tea, coffee (up to 3 cups per day) and herbal teas.

9 **If you are taking medication**, always discuss with your GP before making changes in your diet, particularly when reducing your carbohydrate intake so that any medication you are taking can be adjusted as your health improves.

CARBS *in* FOODS (g/100g)

White rice	78
Sultanas	75
Dates	75
Pasta	72
Brown rice	71
Oats	60
White bread	45
Chapatti	41
Rye bread	39
Brown bread	38
Quinoa	21
Puy lentils	18
Parsnip	18
Cashew	18
Potato	18
Chick peas	14
Turnip	12
Blackberries	10
Avocado	9
Cauliflower	5
Almonds	4
Spinach	4
Pork chop	0
Lamb leg	0
Chicken thigh	0

Counting the CARBS *in* DRINKS

	Serving size	Carbs
Americano – black	340ml (12fl oz)	0g
Americano – milk	340ml (12fl oz)	3g
Americano - cream	340ml (12fl oz)	0g
Cappuccino	340ml (12fl oz)	11g
Latte	340ml (12fl oz)	15g
Hot chocolate	340ml (12fl oz)	39g
Fizzy water	284ml (10fl oz)	0g
Lemonade	284ml (10fl oz)	16g
Orange juice	150ml (5fl oz)	16g
Cola	284ml (10fl oz)	31g
Sweet cider	568ml (1 pint)	24g
Dry cider	568ml (1 pint)	15g
Lager	568ml (1 pint)	12g
Wkd vodka blue	275ml (9½fl oz)	36g
Champagne	125ml (4fl oz)	2g
Dry white wine	250ml (9fl oz)	2g
Red wine	250ml (9fl oz)	1g

PROTEIN
food for strength & structure

Just as a house is built of bricks, a body is built of amino acids which come from proteins including meat, fish, eggs, dairy, pulses (lentils, beans etc), nuts, seeds and soya. Protein is required for the growth and repair of muscle mass, bone strength and healthy organs. Our DNA, immune system and neurotransmitters, such as serotonin (the happy hormone), are also made from amino acids, explaining why a healthy protein intake affects not just our physical bodies but also our mood and wellbeing.

The minimum recommended daily protein intake is 0.8g per kg of bodyweight, and higher levels can be beneficial (some studies show double this level). This equates to at least 56g (2oz) for an average woman (70kg/11 stone) or 67g (2⅓ oz) for an average man (83.6kg/13 stone).

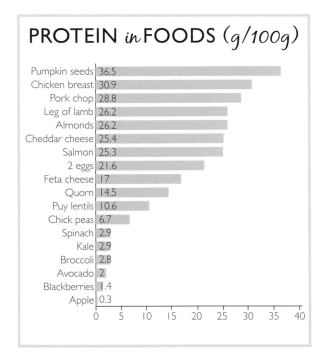

PROTEIN *in* FOODS (g/100g)

Food	Protein (g)
Pumpkin seeds	36.5
Chicken breast	30.9
Pork chop	28.8
Leg of lamb	26.2
Almonds	26.2
Cheddar cheese	25.4
Salmon	25.3
2 eggs	21.6
Feta cheese	17
Quorn	14.5
Puy lentils	10.6
Chick peas	6.7
Spinach	2.9
Kale	2.9
Broccoli	2.8
Avocado	2
Blackberries	1.4
Apple	0.3

Protein portion sizes

We recommend enjoying 100–150g (3½–5½oz) portions of high protein foods, up to three times a day. Two to three medium eggs equate to one portion. The chart above shows the amount of protein in different foods.

Good-quality protein is a key part of your low-carb plan – here is how you can achieve sufficient protein intake:

● **Enjoy a portion of meat,** fish, eggs, dairy, pulses, nuts, seeds or soya with every meal. You can bump up protein by mixing sources, adding a handful of nuts to a chicken salad for instance.

● **Don't fear red meat or eggs** – they are excellent sources of protein.

● **Try to vary your protein** so that you eat each type only once per day. For example, you might have eggs for breakfast, lentils for lunch and meat or fish for dinner.

● **If you are restricting your protein intake,** by following a vegan diet for instance, you may have to repeat protein types across the course of the day. If your protein intake is severely restricted, you could also consider taking protein supplements to maintain good health. If you are worried you are not getting enough protein from your diet, then consult a doctor or qualified dietitian for advice.

● **Try to avoid processed meat products** – the protein content is often reduced, and calories bumped up with carbs. For example, breaded chicken has a third less protein than roast lamb, a similar level of fat and adds bulk by adding lots of carbs. Roast lamb is also exceptionally tasty and satisfying!

● **Eat sausages and bacon in moderation;** try to buy high-meat-content sausages (more than 95% meat) as otherwise you may well be consuming hidden carbs as low-quality sausages are often bulked up with grains like wheat.

● **Higher animal welfare is a consideration** for many people, for both ethical and environmental reasons. If this is you, make friends with a local farm shop or butcher. Ask questions about how the meat is raised; anyone interested in animal welfare will appreciate your interest and this should reassure you that they are sourcing conscientiously.

● If you are worried about the environmental impact of animal foods, please watch Allan Savory's TED talk "How to fight desertification and reverse climate change". Well-managed livestock are an essential element of regenerative farming and protecting the planet.

HEALTHY FATS *for metabolic, brain & hormonal health*

One of the travesties of the low-fat messaging that has dominated food marketing over the last 40 years is that we have been encouraged to avoid delicious and nutritious fats that are essential for our health. Fats build healthy brains and nervous systems (your brain is 60 per cent fat), flexible cell membranes and help produce sex hormones and the stress hormone cortisol. Fats deliver fat-soluble vitamins like vitamins A, D, E and K. Some fats are essential, meaning that we have to eat them as our bodies can't make them. These include the omega-3 fats, such as fish oils, which help to reduce inflammation in the body. When eating low carb, fats become our body's favourite source of fuel for energy.

Enjoy natural fats in food to satiety, and flex your intake depending on your weight-loss goals. If, for example, you are happy with your weight and aiming to consume 2,000 calories on a moderate low-carb plan, your daily fat intake could be up to 160g (5¾oz) per day. If you are aiming to lose weight, then you would be far less generous with added fat and restrict your intake to around 50g (1¾oz) of total fat per day (this equates to around 1,000 calories on a moderate low-carb plan).

This obviously varies depending on many factors (age, sex, activity levels and metabolism) but serves to give you a helpful guide.

"Fat doesn't make you fat" is now a common mantra in the media – here is how to make healthy fat choices:
● **Not all fats are equal** – avoid refined and seed oils, such as sunflower, and margarines which are highly refined and processed. These polyunsaturated fats oxidize when heated, contributing to inflammation in your body.
● **Avoid fats combined with sugar** – doughnuts and cakes are not OK! The fat/sugar combo is the worst as high insulin levels drive fat storage.
● **Avoid low-fat products** – these tend to be bulked up with carbs.
● **Enjoy dairy products**, which are an excellent source of healthy fats and may help to improve cardiovascular health.
● **Plump for fattier versions of meat** which are tasty and usually more economical, such as mince, beef shin and lamb neck.
● **Cook with lard, butter and coconut oil** – these saturated fats are stable when heated. Olive oil

> "High insulin levels promote fat storage & impair your ability to burn body fat as fuel"

can be used cold in salads or gently heated – it is a monounsaturated fat and is also protected by antioxidants. Animal fats, such as duck fat, which can be left over from a roast, are also heat stable for cooking.
● **Eat oily fish** for essential omega-3 at least twice a week – choose sardines, mackerel, trout, salmon or anchovies.

How does eating fat affect weight loss?
It may sound paradoxical to eat more fat when you are trying to lose weight. We have been led to believe that fats, especially the saturated versions, are bad for us and cause us to be overweight. But the evidence shows that higher fat diets can lead to significant weight loss.

The fats that we recommend you avoid are the modern refined and heavily processed oils which come from seeds like sunflower – otherwise known as polyunsaturated oils. These oils oxidize when they are heated and so are less healthy. You will find they are widely used in industrial food production, usually alongside lots of refined carbohydrates, as well as promoted for cooking.

Natural fats from meat, fish, dairy, eggs, nuts and whole seeds have been eaten by humans since the beginning of time. As well as being tasty, they provide an excellent fuel when you start eating low carb.

Interestingly, eating more fat is a useful strategy to lose weight, maintain weight or even gain weight. What differs between these goals is how much food is eaten.

To lose weight, you need to burn the fat calories that you are wearing around your middle. When insulin levels are low (from eating low carb), your body can relearn to switch between burning the fat calories that you eat and those you have previously stored. The exciting thing is that you feel less hungry, unlike when following a low-calorie or low-fat diet. A low-calorie diet is usually based on eating refined carbs and restricting fat, hence spiking blood sugar and insulin levels even in healthy people. High insulin levels promote fat storage and impair your ability to burn body fat as fuel.

A groundbreaking study in 2018 measured the total energy expenditure across three diets – low, moderate and high carb (20 per cent, 40 per cent and 60 per cent of calories respectively). The study methodology was robust, using a randomized trial where the food intake was controlled by providing meals to the 164 participants. Reducing carbohydrate intake significantly increased metabolism – those on the low-carb diet utilized an additional 209 calories compared to those on the highest carb diet.

BECOMING A FAT BURNER
the secret of eating less

Have you ever treated yourself to a cooked breakfast, maybe at the weekend or on holiday as a treat, and been surprised that you could go through most of the day without thinking about food? This is very common and underlines my point. When we eat more satisfying meals, such as a cooked breakfast containing protein and fat from the eggs and bacon, we feel fuller for longer and don't need to snack all the time.

Not snacking between meals is known as intermittent fasting and is another way to help your body to burn the calories from stored body fat as energy. With low-carb foods you are able to switch relatively easily to burning fat because your insulin levels are relatively

low (insulin is a fat-storage hormone). There are many benefits to fasting – from losing weight, to improving your immunity and longevity. It also reduces the amount of time you need to think about or prepare food.

Here are some tips for how to experiment with intermittent fasting:
● **Firstly, restrict yourself to a 12-hour eating window,** say from 7am to 7pm, so that you enjoy a 12-hour overnight fast. This benefits your metabolism as rather than constantly digesting food your body can focus on other functions.
● **Then try to focus on enjoying just three meals a day,** with 5–6 hours between each meal and no snacks. This is known as intermittent fasting as between meals you will be able to burn body fat for energy rather than using the calories from food. This may be sufficient for you to lose weight, provided that your blood sugar and insulin levels are stable.
● **As you gain control of your appetite**, you may choose to occasionally miss a meal, or replace a meal with a low-carb snack instead. Enjoying coffee with cream, snacking on some olives, nuts or an egg, or sipping chicken broth can rev up your fat burning and quickly send food cravings packing.

Fasting can have extremely good results for many people, not just for weight loss but generally improving many health markers. If you wish to delve further into this area, look up the work of Dr Jason Fung who has many books and YouTube videos to his name.

Eating less often allows you to eat delicious, nutritious meals to control your food intake, without hunger or a drop in energy levels, and achieve your weight-loss goals. Intermittent fasting is safe for people with type 2 diabetes, provided that you have discussed medication with your GP.

> "When we eat more satisfying meals, such as a cooked breakfast containing protein & fat from the eggs & bacon, we feel fuller for longer and don't need to snack all the time"

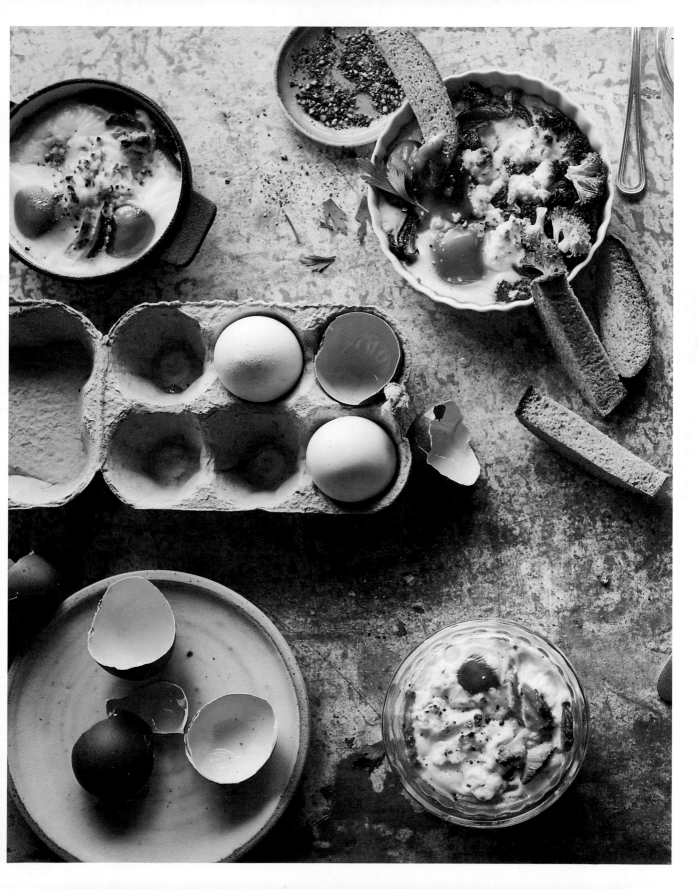

Weekly
MEAL PLANS

Here are two meal plans – one for weight loss and the other designed to work as a maintenance plan once you've lost weight.

Both these plans are low carb and the main meals are mostly the same. You will see that the maintenance plan has added extras, such as a glass of wine at the weekend or sometimes a dessert. This is because when you're not trying to lose weight you can generally eat more calories. Think quality of food first, then adjust your portion sizes and extras to meet your own health and weight-loss goals.

If you are not overweight, prediabetic or diabetic, and therefore more liberal low carb (see the CarbScale – page 29), then you may do perfectly well including a limited amount of higher carb foods occasionally but make these the exception rather than the rule.

We haven't included snacks, simply because in our experience people do very well on three meals a day, or less if you are also practising intermittent fasting. But if you do feel that you need a snack, then try to keep that low carb too. You might grab some olives, an avocado, a boiled egg or a handful of nuts and berries.

Many of the recipes are multi-purpose or ideal for batch cooking, such as the Quichata on page 86, Whipped Chicken Liver Pâté on page 158, Quick Ragù on page 121 or Hülya's Aubergines on page 169. Cook them once, store in the fridge and use them for different meals throughout the week.

To take to work, try the Beetburgers on page 146, the Peppers & Sardines on page 132, the Feta & Herb Mini Frittatas on page 95, or butter a Quick Brown Bread Bap from page 110 and fill it with chicken, ham or grated carrot and tahini.

Weight-loss meal plan

	BREAKFAST	LUNCH	DINNER	DRINKS	TIP FOR THE DAY
MON	Coffee with 1 tablespoon of cream (skip breakfast)	Peppers & Sardines (page 132) with a mixed salad	Quichata (page 86) and Green Salad (page 57)	Water, tea, coffee	Take a brisk 25-minute walk
TUES	Simple Scrambled Eggs (page 98)	Grilled Paneer & Broccoli Traybake (page 144)	Quick Ragù on Savoy Pezzi (page 121)	Water, tea, coffee	Swim, cycle or just walk
WEDS	Coffee with 1 tablespoon of cream (skip breakfast)	Leftover Quichata (page 86) and Green Salad (page 57)	Salmon with Thyme, Orange & Fennel (page 137)	Water, tea, coffee	Attend an exercise class or go for a walk
THURS	Cheese & Ham Omelette (page 83)	Leftover Salmon with Thyme, Orange & Fennel (page 137)	Sausage and Halloumi Kebabs or Traybake (page 161)	Water, tea, coffee	Take a brisk 25-minute walk
FRI	Greek yogurt & berries or Strawberry & Lemon Yogurt (page 75)	Beetburgers & Avocado Salsa (page 146)	Sea Bass with Tarragon (page 138)	Water, tea, coffee	Dance, run upstairs a few times or attend an exercise class
SAT	BRUNCH Mushroom Rarebit with Poached Eggs (page 84)		Steak & Chips (page 112) with green vegetables	Water, tea, coffee	Get out into nature and move your body
SUN	Coffee with 1 tablespoon of cream (skip breakfast)	Gammon Steak, Parsley & Leek Cream (page 125) with steamed broccoli	Chilean Chorizo Soup (page 106)	Water, tea, coffee	Make a shopping list for the week ahead – get prepared

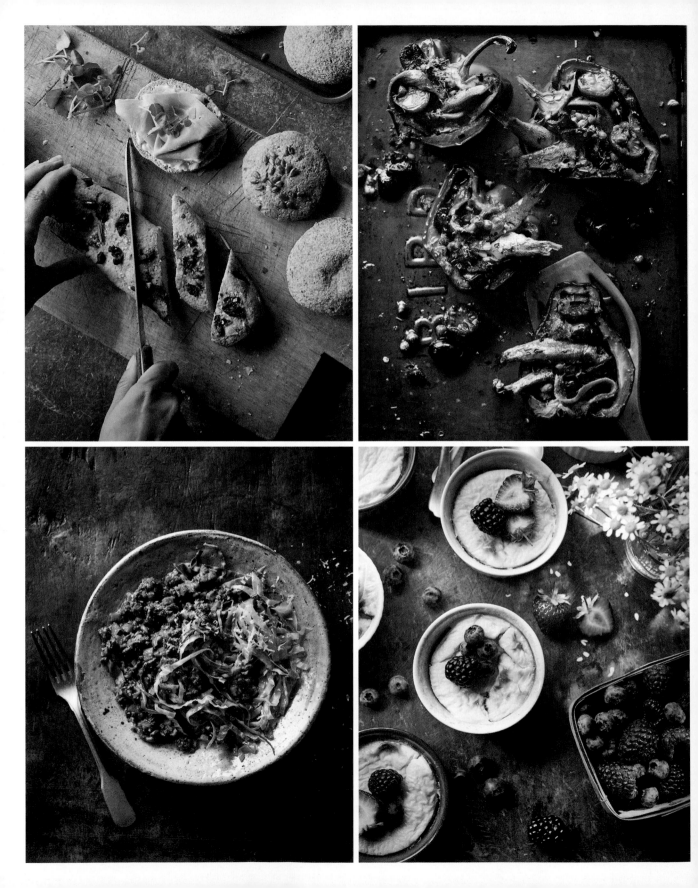

Maintenance meal plan

	BREAKFAST	LUNCH	DINNER	DRINKS	TIP FOR THE DAY
MON	Sasha's Salad (page 58)	Peppers & Sardines (page 132) with a mixed salad 2 squares of 85% dark chocolate	Quichata (page 86) with Steamed Vegetables (page 128) Baked Fruit & Coconut Custard (page 184)	Water, tea, coffee	Take a brisk 25-minute walk
TUES	Simple Scrambled Eggs (page 98) with Quick Brown Bread Bap (page 110)	Grilled Paneer & Broccoli Traybake (page 144)	Quick Ragù on Savoy Pezzi (page 121) Giancarlo's Gorgeous Raspberry Cream (page 181)	Water, tea, coffee	Swim, cycle or just walk
WEDS	Coffee with 1 tablespoon of cream (skip breakfast)	Leftover Quichata (page 86) and Green Salad (page 57) 2 squares of 85% dark chocolate	Salmon with Thyme, Orange & Fennel (page 137)	Water, tea, coffee	Attend an exercise class or go for a walk
THURS	Cheese & Ham Omelette (page 83)	Leftover Salmon with Thyme, Orange & Fennel (page 137)	Sausage and Halloumi Kebabs or Traybake (page 161)	Water, tea, coffee	Take a brisk 25-minute walk
FRI	Your choice from 5 Ways with Yogurt (pages 74–77)	Beetburgers & Avocado Salsa (page 146)	Sea Bass with Tarragon (page 134) Baked Cheesecake with Summer Berries (page 176)	1 gin & reduced-sugar tonic or 175ml (6fl oz) glass of wine	Dance, run upstairs a few times or attend an exercise class
SAT	Your choice from 5 Ways with Yogurt (pages 74–77)	Mushroom Rarebit with Poached Eggs (page 84)	Steak & Chips (page 112) with green vegetables Blueberry & Lemon Ice Cream (page 174)	1 gin & reduced-sugar tonic or 175ml (6fl oz) glass of wine	Get out into nature and move your body
SUN	Your choice of eggs, eg Boursin Baked Eggs (page 94)	Gammon Steak, Parsley & Leek Cream (page 121) with steamed broccoli	Chilean Chorizo Soup (page 106) with Quick Brown Bread Bap (page 110)	Water, tea, coffee	Make a shopping list for the week ahead – get prepared

GOING & STAYING LOW CARB

Dr Jen Unwin, Chartered Clinical and Health Psychologist

There is absolutely no doubt in my mind how effective low-carb diets can be for people both physically and mentally. I've seen the evidence in myself, my family members, patients and people online. I've read the journal articles and looked at the evidence. Most of us know when we are eating too much, especially when it comes to sugary, carb-heavy treats. The answer to many of our health and wellbeing issues comes down to following just one simple piece of advice: eliminate sugar and refined carbohydrates from your diet. That's it. Simple, yes but not easy. Why is this one rule so hard to follow consistently and what effective tips are there for succeeding?

SUGAR *addiction*

There is plenty of evidence that sugar and junk food act on our brains much like other addictive substances such as alcohol or nicotine. The reward centre lights up when we eat carb-heavy foods, releasing the feel-good neurotransmitters dopamine and serotonin. Dopamine is linked to motivation and reward and your brain will drive you to repeat the experience that triggers it. Over time though, the more you consume sugar, the more the brain adjusts by reducing the number of dopamine receptors, so you need to eat more and more to get the same effect. At the same time, you lose interest in other activities and focus increasingly on food. Serotonin is the comfort neurotransmitter and is made from tryptophan in the brain. Usually, tryptophan competes with other molecules to enter the brain but in the presence of insulin (the hormone released when we eat sugar or the starchy carbs that digest down into sugar, see page 7) it enters the brain in greater amounts, meaning more serotonin. If this is repeated too often, tryptophan is depleted and so serotonin production is reduced. Eventually, less serotonin means fewer

happy hormones. The whole thing is a tragic trap. Sugar consumption leads to the release of dopamine and serotonin but repeated too often this means a reduction in the availability of those substances in the brain, leading to reduced motivation and happiness (sometimes described as brain fog), leading to more cravings for sugary foods and the temporary boost they deliver.

Like other addictive processes, we often know that we should cut down on sugar and carbs as they are harming our physical and mental health, but yet struggle to do so. Our brains have been hijacked at a very fundamental, primitive level and this trumps the logical thinking part of them. We are evolutionarily programmed to pursue sugary and sweet foods to avoid winter starvation. This is partly why giving up sugar is so challenging. We live in perpetual feast and store mode.

Sugar is the first psychoactive drug we are given as children. Most of us will have very happy memories of childhood sweets, ice cream and puddings. Some families, like mine and Katie's, enjoyed food as a major part of the day, with carbohydrates and sugar taking centre stage on the altar! One of my earliest memories is of making cheese scones at Sunday school and

> "There is plenty of evidence that sugar & junk food act on our brains much like other addictive substances such as alcohol or nicotine"

eating them warm, slathered in butter. I had a serious sweet habit, even to the point of buying family bags of Minstrels on the way home from school and eating the lot. Some food addiction specialists consider sugar to be a gateway drug, because we encounter it so young. Caffeine, nicotine and alcohol tend to come into our lives when we are somewhat older. Have you noticed that people who give up cigarettes and alcohol often develop a really sweet tooth and put on weight? It's because the brain is trying to get its dopamine and serotonin fix from another source. It's easier, I would argue, to avoid cigarettes and alcohol than to avoid sugar, because we have to eat, it's everywhere, and in so many processed foods. Not only that, but there are "pushers" at every turn. The office cupcake baker, kindly relatives making puddings and treats, people buying us chocolates as a "thank you", even charities organizing cake sales.

In addition to its addictive qualities, our culture has normalized the excessive consumption of sugar and carbohydrate in recent decades. It's everywhere and every day. Cereal for breakfast, snacks morning, afternoon and evening, sandwiches for lunch, pasta for tea, smoothies, juices and lattes. Birthdays, Easter, Christmas, Valentine's Day, Mother's Day, holidays, anniversaries and weekends are all excuses to "treat yourself". We are bombarded with temptation at work, at the garage, in the supermarkets and at checkouts. It's a miracle that anyone achieves a normal weight and metabolism.

So, my message is, don't think of yourself as having no willpower and don't berate yourself if you have found quitting sugar and carbs hard. It is! And it isn't your fault. We are at the mercy of our biology and our modern culture. But knowledge is power, and freedom is possible. Many thousands have achieved it and you can too.

> "We often know that we should cut down on sugar & carbs as they are harming our physical & mental health, but yet struggle to do so"

Your passport TO FREEDOM FROM SUGAR

Come with me now on a journey to freedom from sugar and carbs!

Every good journey starts with a lot of thinking, dreaming and planning, so that's where we will begin. The most important thing to consider in some detail is: where are you heading? What is your dream destination? Otherwise, you won't know when you get there or how to get back on course if you take a diversion (which you will!). It's a long day on the golf course if you don't know where the hole is, as a colleague of mine used to say!

What will life look like when you have mastered low-carb living? What will you be doing that you are not doing now? What will you be feeling about yourself? What will other people notice about you? What opportunities might arise?

Giving up sugar and carbs will be tough at times, so what is at the end of the rainbow to keep you pushing through, getting up and trying again?

If you find yourself saying "I'll have lost weight", or "I'll have reversed my diabetes", try to dig deeper to think what difference that will make. What will be different because you have achieved those things? For example, how will you feel? What will you be doing? If I was making a documentary about you, what would the final episode show you doing and saying? People often say things like, "I'll be able to play with the grandchildren", or "I want to enjoy my retirement", or "I'd love to feel good about how I look".

The next job is packing. What are you taking on your journey? We all have unique strengths and talents that we bring to the many challenges of home and work life. Think about the things you are naturally good at or that have been part of successfully dealing with previous challenges. For me, it would be my organizational skills and single-mindedness once I make a decision. Also, who are you taking with you? Is there someone or even a few people who might support and help you on this journey? Your cheerleaders. Hopefully someone in your household will come on the same journey. Support is an essential part of this process. If there isn't anyone nearby, join an online group, such as www.facebook.com/lowcarbtogether or www.lowcarbprogram.com.

Imagine in a year's time that you are approaching your dream destination. What or who is it that helped you along the way? How did you do it? Pack up your best self, your support team and let's go!

It's a long journey you are going on, so there will be many, many stopping off points. What will be your first port of call? We are all different, start at different points, travel at different speeds, have different destinations, and so have different first steps. What would tell you that you are, for example, one tenth of the way there? There is no right answer. For some it is giving up sugar in tea and coffee (no more adding sugar to things), for some there might be a specific food they need to quit, such as biscuits or bread. Another approach is to not focus on giving things up but adding them in. For example, starting the day with protein-based breakfasts instead of cereal, taking a healthy low-carb lunch to work or pre-preparing tasty protein-based evening meals. When you've reached your first staging post and had a little rest there, move on to the next and so on. If you try something and it doesn't suit you, go another way. There are many roads to the same destination.

Your last job is to keep some sort of a record of your journey. This will encourage you to notice all the good things that happen along the way and work out which strategies work well for you. Some people like to get weighed. Try not to do this more than once a week. Measuring around your tummy in the same place once a week is also great feedback. Also, what about keeping a mood rating out of 10 each day, or an energy rating? You may feel a bit ropey for the first week of cutting down sugar and carbohydrates but after that should notice more mental and physical wellbeing. Maybe take photos in the same clothes once a month? What else do you notice along the way? Fewer headaches, better skin, better sleep? Noticing all these successes will encourage you onward and will also serve as a reminder of all the benefits if you have a wobble.

Establishing new habits is key to long-term success. The low-carb lifestyle needs to be sustainable for you and this will not be achieved by willpower alone (or you would have already succeeded). I heard someone say recently that it should be called "won't power" not willpower because actually we are trying not to act on the impulses from our primitive brains. Rather we need to engage our thinking brains so they tell us "I could eat that biscuit, but I won't because I want to reach my dream destination and I feel better without it".

Enjoy the trip!

"Establishing new habits is key to long-term success. The low-carb lifestyle needs to be sustainable for you & this will not be achieved by willpower alone"

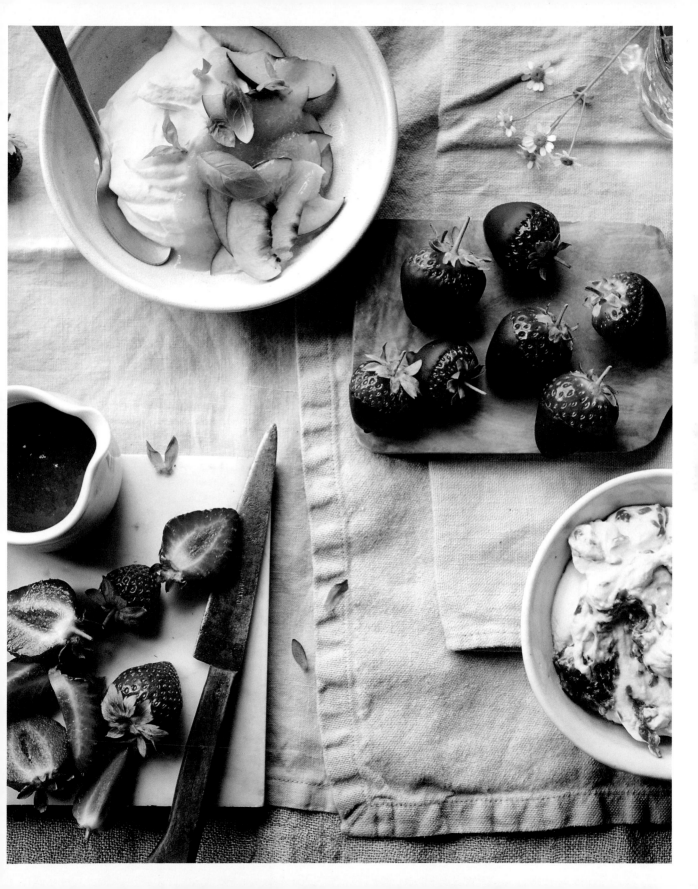

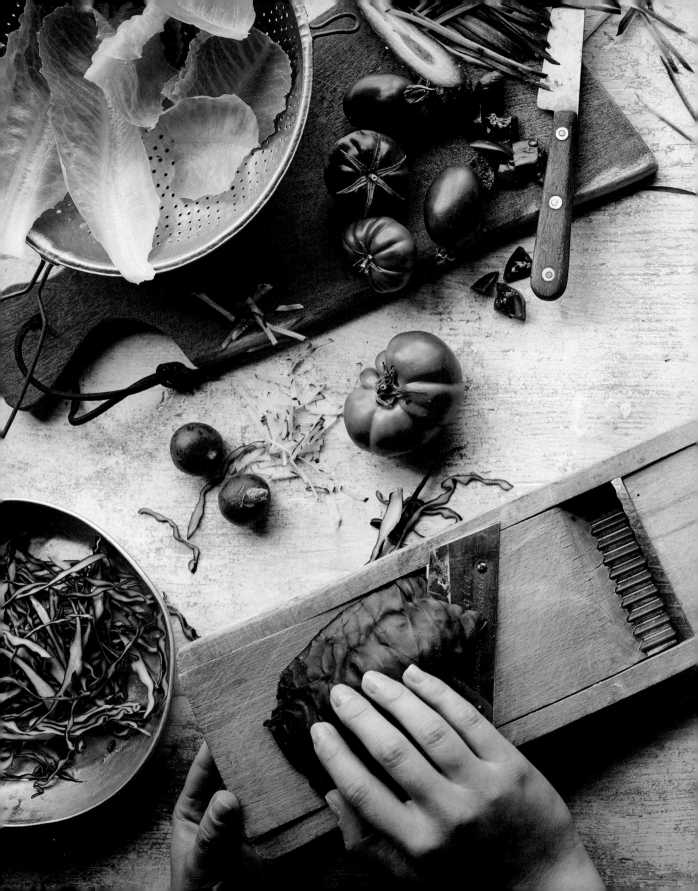

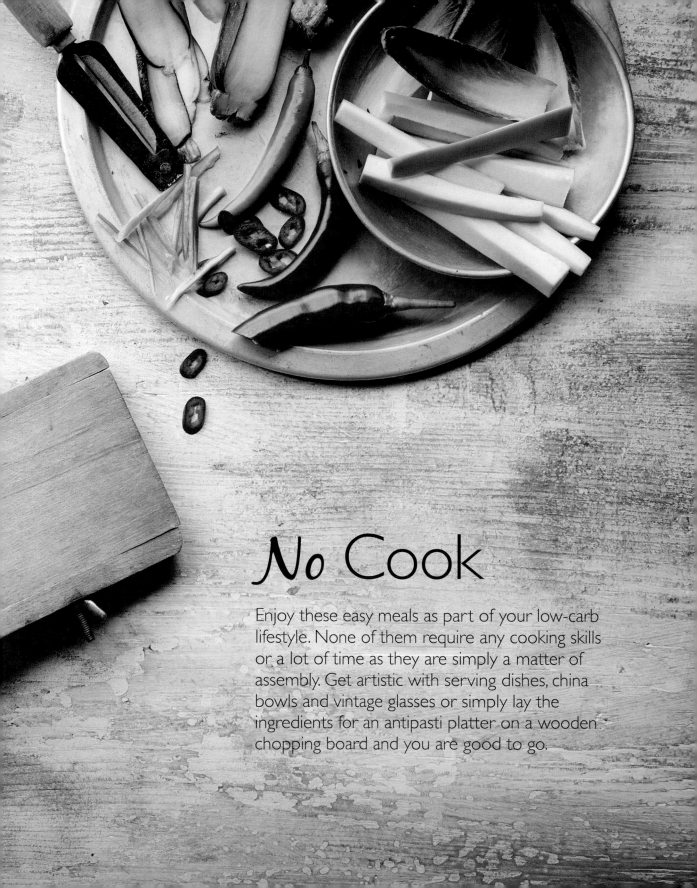

No Cook

Enjoy these easy meals as part of your low-carb lifestyle. None of them require any cooking skills or a lot of time as they are simply a matter of assembly. Get artistic with serving dishes, china bowls and vintage glasses or simply lay the ingredients for an antipasti platter on a wooden chopping board and you are good to go.

French Assiette

SERVES 4

For the celeriac remoulade

3 tablespoons mayonnaise

2 tablespoons full-fat Greek yogurt

1 heaped tablespoon Dijon or
   wholegrain mustard

juice of ½ lemon

300g (10½oz) celeriac, peeled

salt and freshly ground black pepper

To serve (optional)

200g (7oz) pâté

12 slices of cold, cooked ham

8 small gherkins

12 radishes

16 caper berries

4 soft-boiled eggs

a large handful of watercress

4 round tomatoes

2 chicory or Little Gem lettuces

Per serving of celeriac remoulade
7g net carbs, 1.5g fibre, 2g protein,
5g fat, 83kcal

This recipe is inspired by a visit to a restaurant in France where to start the meal guests were served a simple dressed green salad and huge jars of homemade pickled gherkins and vegetables. Enormous slabs of pâté, cold ham and celeriac remoulade were brought to the table and everyone helped themselves. I loved it and have recreated it here with simple shop-bought items that often get overlooked, such as gherkins, radishes and caper berries. Other delicious additions are soft-boiled eggs, cold cuts, watercress, tomatoes and chicory or small lettuce leaves for holding the pâté and remoulade. Use any leftover celeriac in the Mash on page 117 or in the Creamy Vegetable Soup on page 107.

Mix the mayonnaise, yogurt, mustard and lemon juice together in a bowl. Coarsely grate the celeriac over the top (or do this in a food processor for speed). Stir through and add seasoning as necessary. Serve in a small bowl with any of the additions suggested. The remoulade will keep in the fridge for a couple of days.

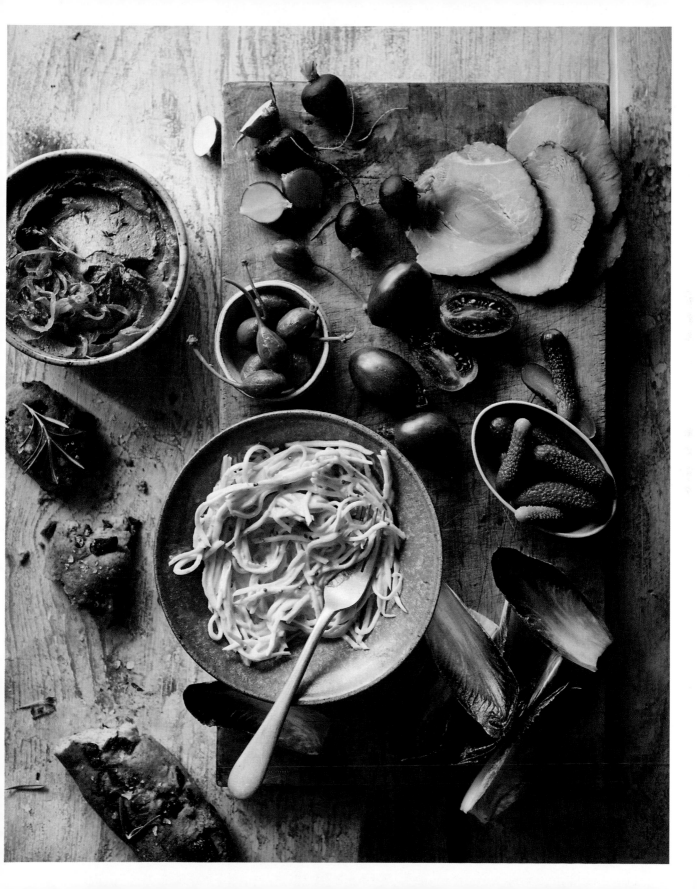

Chicken, Apple & Dill Salad

SERVES 2

zest and juice of ½ lemon

4 level tablespoons thick Greek yogurt

2 cooked chicken breasts, weighing about 240g (8½oz), shredded

1 tablespoon dill, roughly chopped

1 small apple, unpeeled and roughly chopped

1 heart of celery or 2 celery sticks with leaves, finely chopped

2 tablespoons extra virgin olive oil

2 teaspoons red wine vinegar

4 firm lettuce leaves, such as Romaine, or 6 Little Gem leaves

salt and freshly ground black pepper

Per serving 11g net carbs, 4g fibre, 40g protein, 22g fat, 417kcal

The celery leaves are key to this salad as something magical happens when you use them with apple and dill; this humble dish becomes more than the sum of its parts. The idea is to spoon some of the lemon yogurt on to a leaf then top it with the salad. This is a brunch or light meal in our house, and it can be bumped up with the addition of soft-boiled eggs or a warm, buttered Bap (page 110). The salad keeps in the fridge for a couple of days. If you have your own cooked chicken, it is better than one bought ready-cooked as they can contain starches, which increase the carbs. Leftover dill can be used in the New Russian Salad on page 70 and the Snow White Salad on page 63.

Mix the lemon zest and juice together with the yogurt in a small bowl and season to taste. Divide it in two and spoon it into a pile on 2 shallow bowls or plates.

Mix the remaining ingredients, apart from the lettuce, together and season to taste. Transfer to the 2 bowls, laying it next to the lemon yogurt, and serve with the lettuce on the side.

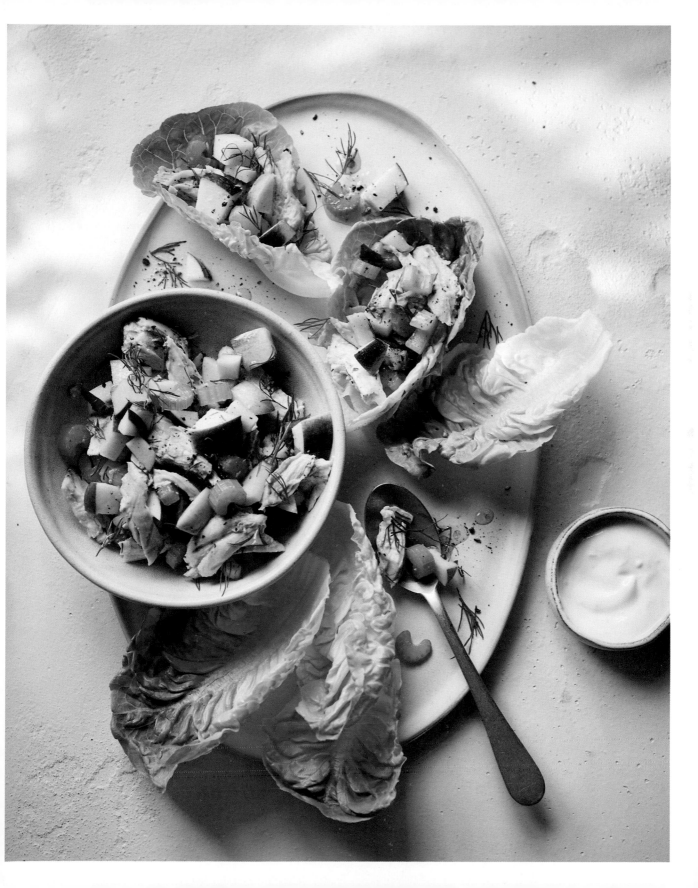

Italian Antipasti Board

SERVES 4

For the Caprese salad

300g (10½oz) flavourful, ripe tomatoes

2 x 125g (4½oz) buffalo
  mozzarella balls

20 fresh basil leaves

½ teaspoon dried oregano

3 tablespoons best-quality extra
  virgin olive oil

salt and freshly ground black pepper

To serve (optional)

16 slices of salami

20 olives

1 jar of marinated mushrooms,
  artichokes or peppers

Focaccia Sticks (page 110)

Per serving of Caprese salad
3.5g net carbs, 1g fibre, 15g protein,
26g fat, 301kcal

We like to rustle up this display of Italian goodies when we're hungry and have no time to cook. The classic Italian tomato and mozzarella salad, Insalata Caprese, should really only be made when tomatoes are sweet and flavourful. My favourites are the large misshapen Cuore di Bue (oxheart) or Marmande varieties. Failing that, heirloom tomatoes look beautiful and have fantastic flavour. If you can, use buffalo mozzarella and your best extra virgin olive oil. Optional additions to the salad include salami, olives, jars of marinated vegetables in oil and one of our Focaccia Sticks (page 110).

Cut the tomatoes into 1cm- (½in-) thick slices or quarter them if small. Slice the mozzarella into 1cm- (½in-) thick slices or tear into thick shreds.

Lay the tomato slices on a wooden chopping board or carving dish (preferably with a groove to catch the juices). Season with a little salt and pepper. Tear over the basil leaves. Now lay over the mozzarella, season again, then scatter over the oregano and drizzle over the olive oil.

Serve straight away with any additions you like.

Salmon Poke Bowl

SERVES 1

160g (5¾oz) very fresh salmon or
  yellowfin tuna, cut into 1.5cm
  (⅝in) dice

2 spring onions, finely chopped

a small handful of coriander,
  tough stems removed

½ avocado, cut into 1.5cm (⅝in) dice

1 tablespoon toasted black or white
  sesame seeds

¼–½ red chilli, very finely diced

For the tamari dressing

½ teaspoon wasabi paste or
  English mustard

juice of ½ lime

2 tablespoons tamari or dark or
  light soy sauce

1 teaspoon toasted sesame oil

1 teaspoon finely grated fresh ginger

Per serving 9.8g net carbs, 6.9g fibre,
38.8g protein, 38.7g fat, 558kcal

Poke, pronounced "pokay", originally comes from Hawaii and means "to slice", referring to the way the fish is cut so that it soaks up the dressing quickly. It is crucial to find sashimi-grade salmon or tuna, or previously commercially frozen fish, as it is eaten raw. Wipe the cut lime over the leftover avocado half, then keep it in the fridge for a day or two.

Combine the wasabi, lime juice, tamari, oil and ginger in a bowl. Adjust the flavours to suit your taste – it should have bite from the wasabi and sourness from the lime. It won't look like a lot, but it is just to coat the fish and avocado, not to swamp it.

Combine the salmon, spring onions and coriander in a bowl. Pour the dressing over the top, add the avocado and gently stir to combine. Scatter over sesame seeds and chilli and serve straight away.

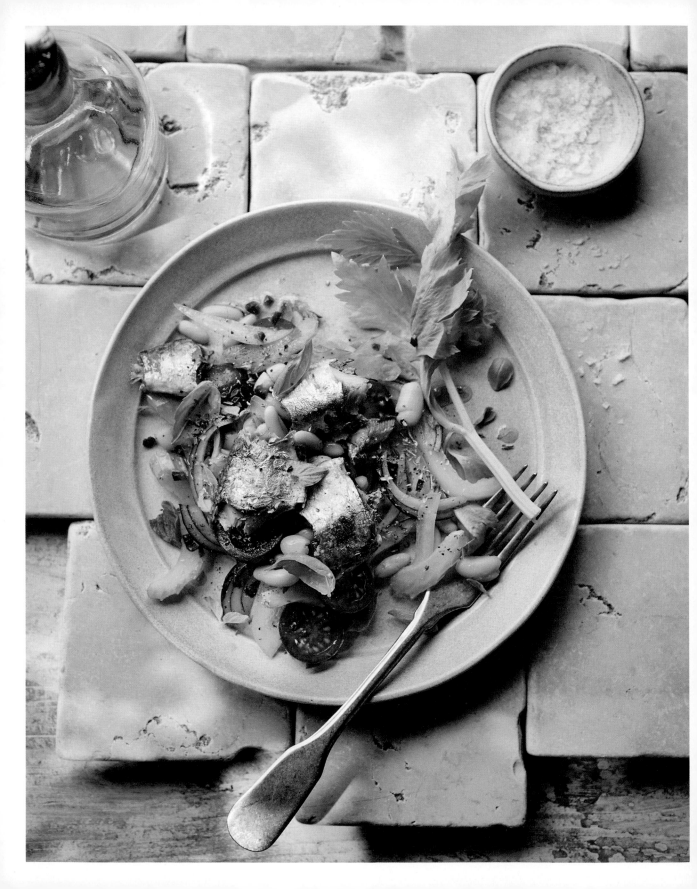

Sardines with Cannellini Beans & Celery

SERVES 4

1 red onion, thinly sliced into half-moons

10 cherry tomatoes, halved

2 celery sticks, cut finely on the
    diagonal, plus a small handful of
    celery leaves, to garnish

1 small yellow pepper, cut into thin strips

240g (8½oz) cooked or canned
    cannellini or borlotti beans, drained

1 tablespoon fresh oregano leaves or
    ½ teaspoon dried oregano

a little finely chopped red chilli, to taste,
    or ¼ teaspoon chilli flakes

2 tablespoons red wine vinegar

5 tablespoons extra virgin olive oil

2 x 120g (4½oz) cans sardines in
    olive oil, drained (170g/6oz net weight)

a small handful of basil leaves

salt and freshly ground black pepper

Per serving 14g net carbs, 4.8g fibre,
14g protein, 22g fat, 326kcal

When Giancarlo was growing up in rural Tuscany, he rarely saw a fresh fish as he lived too far from the sea. So, salted fish, such as herrings or sardines, or jars of tuna in oil sold at the local market were a real treat. He often tells our children that one suppertime, as the youngest in the family, he was simply given the "smell" of a canned and salted herring. His father wiped the fish over a piece of bread and Giancarlo had to be happy with that while the adults shared the fish.

A simple combination of cooked beans, canned tuna and onions is commonplace on the Tuscan table. We like to use canned sardines as they are sustainable, economical and just as nutritious as their fresh counterparts. If you want to reduce the carbs switch the beans for soft-boiled eggs or toasted nuts.

Put the sliced onions in a bowl of cold water and leave to soak for 10 minutes. (This will make them less potent.) Drain well.

Put the tomatoes, celery, pepper, beans, oregano and chilli in a large bowl, add the onions and mix with a large spoon. Splash over the vinegar and 4 tablespoons of the oil, season with salt and pepper and stir again.

Break the sardines into the salad. Stir gently to combine, without flaking the fish. Taste and add more seasoning or chilli as necessary. (At this point, before adding the basil, the salad will keep well in an airtight container in the fridge for a couple of days.)

To serve, arrange the salad on a large plate. Tear over the basil and celery leaves and drizzle over the remaining olive oil.

Spicy Tuna & Noodle Salad

SERVES 1

2 spring onions, finely chopped

1 packet shirataki or konjac noodles
(approx. 170g/6oz drained weight)

2.5cm (1in) fresh ginger, peeled
and grated

a little finely chopped green or red chilli,
to taste, or a pinch of chilli flakes

juice of ½ lime

1 tablespoon fish sauce

1–2 teaspoons tamari or dark or
light soy sauce

a small bunch of coriander, roughly
chopped, stems finely chopped
(optional)

1 small carrot, scrubbed and grated

100g (3½oz) canned or jarred tuna,
drained weight

1 tablespoon peanuts or toasted black
or white sesame seeds (optional)

Per serving 9.4g net carbs, 14.2g
fibre, 34.8g protein, 5.4g fat, 265kcal

I have a beautifully simple Japanese bowl that I use for this spicy cold salad. I am convinced it alters the taste when you have lovely china to eat from! Adjust the ingredients depending on what you have and finish with the herbs and nuts. Use tuna from a jar or can, either works well, or you can also use salmon if you prefer.

Put the spring onions in a bowl of cold water and leave to soak for 5 minutes to reduce their potency. Rinse the noodles in a sieve in cold water and leave to drain.

Mix the ginger, chilli, lime juice, fish sauce and tamari together in a mixing bowl. Add the coriander, carrot, drained spring onions and noodles and toss through. Then add the tuna and gently stir though. Transfer to a bowl and top with the nuts or seeds, if using.

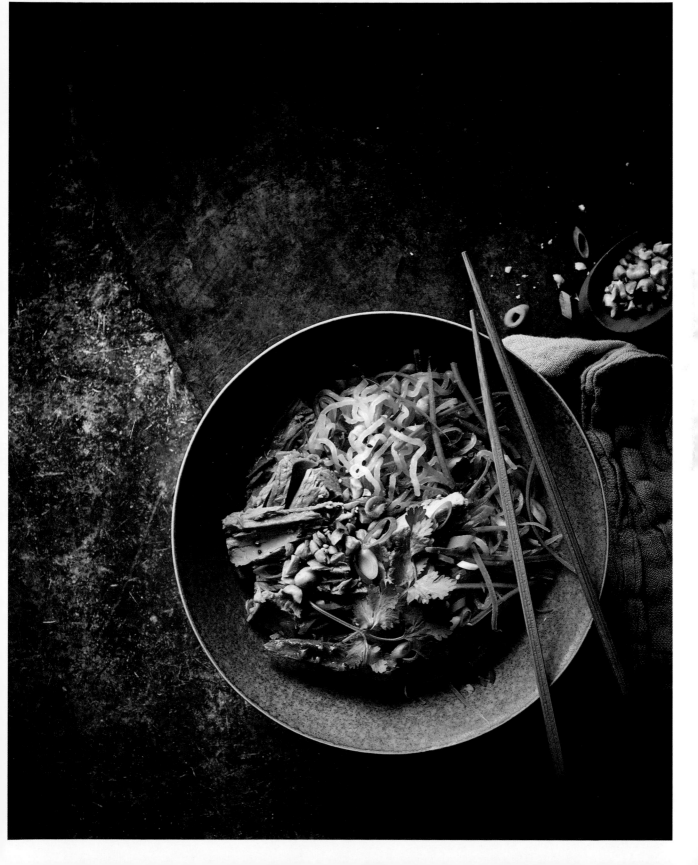

The Big Slaw

SERVES 2

100g (3½oz) carrots, scrubbed and coarsely grated

200g (7oz) red or white cabbage

240g (8½oz) cooked or canned chickpeas, black, borlotti or cannellini beans, drained

1 green chilli or a pinch of chilli flakes

a small handful of coriander or flat-leaf parsley, roughly chopped

1 tablespoon extra virgin olive oil

juice of ½ lemon or a splash of cider vinegar

½ teaspoon ground cumin

½ teaspoon black onion (nigella) seeds

For the tahini dressing

2 tablespoons tahini

juice of ½ lemon or a splash of cider vinegar

salt and freshly ground black pepper

To serve (optional)

4 soft-boiled eggs, halved

1 teaspoon sesame seeds

a handful of toasted nuts, such as almonds, hazelnuts or peanuts, chopped

Per serving of slaw 20g net carbs, 8g fibre, 12.8g protein, 18.5g fat, 367kcal

This simple and filling slaw is perfect throughout the year as it doesn't rely on summer vegetables. I have spiced it up and given it some heat with a dusting of cumin, chilli and one of my favourite spices – black onion seeds, also known as nigella seeds. With the lemon juice and fresh vegetables, it's perfect for boosting your immunity in winter. For extra protein, add a couple of soft-boiled eggs, sesame seeds or toasted nuts. To save time, buy a ready-chopped coleslaw mix. The tangy, nutty dressing is great on roast vegetables or steamed broccoli too. If you want to reduce the carbs, switch the chickpeas or beans for eggs or toasted nuts.

Mix the dressing ingredients together and add 2 tablespoons of water to dilute to a creamy consistency. Season to taste with extra lemon juice, salt and pepper. Use straight away or keep in the fridge for up to 3 days.

Mix all the salad ingredients together in a large bowl. Divide between 2 salad bowls, splash over the dressing and serve.

Green Salad & Vinaigrette

SERVES 4

400g (14oz) green salad leaves, such as round lettuce, chicory, radicchio, rocket and/or watercress

For the vinaigrette

1 tablespoon red wine vinegar

4 tablespoons extra virgin olive oil

1 teaspoon Dijon mustard

salt and freshly ground black pepper

Per serving 1.3g net carbs, 2g fibre, 1.6g protein, 13.8g fat, 138kcal

I am convinced that making vinaigrette got me hooked on cooking at an early age. My mother would ask me to measure one part vinegar to four parts oil in a jar then to shake the ingredients together and watch the vinegar emulsify with the oil. It was my job to taste the dressing and tell her if it needed more acidity or seasoning. My young palate was trained, and she empowered me with a sense that my opinion counted. The dressing keeps in the in the jar in the fridge for up to a week. Remove from the fridge 30 minutes before you need it and shake before serving.

Make a simple salad with one type of leaf or add in bitter notes like chicory or radicchio, sweet herbs such as mint and dill, buttery round or lamb's lettuce, or spicy leaves of rocket or watercress. It all depends on what's in season and in your fridge or garden. In spring, I add foraged leaves of Jack by the Hedge, dandelion and the first herbs of the year.

A green salad is a perfect starter and can stretch a meal out into two courses, giving you more time to feel full. Alternatively serve it on the same plate as roasted meats or fish as the vinaigrette creates a sauce. If your main course already has a sauce, don't mix it; serve the salad in a separate bowl on the side.

Put the vinaigrette ingredients into a jar with a lid and shake to combine. Season to taste. Toss the salad leaves in the dressing just before serving.

Sasha's Salad

SERVES 2

1 avocado, cubed or sliced

*1 large tomato or 6 cherry tomatoes,
cut into bite-sized pieces*

zest and juice of ½ lemon

2 tablespoons extra virgin olive oil

50g (1 ¾oz) feta cheese, crumbled

salt and freshly ground black pepper

Per serving 3.8g net carbs, 3g fibre,
5.5g protein, 34g fat, 351kcal

Sasha is our son's girlfriend and lived with us during lockdown. Most mornings she would make this salad to start the day and it soon became a family favourite; quick to knock up and filling enough to carry you through to lunch. For a vegan version, add a drained can of beans or chickpeas instead of the feta.

Mix the avocado with the tomato, lemon zest and juice, olive oil and salt and pepper in a bowl. Divide between 2 serving bowls, crumble over the feta and eat straight away or keep in the fridge for up to an hour.

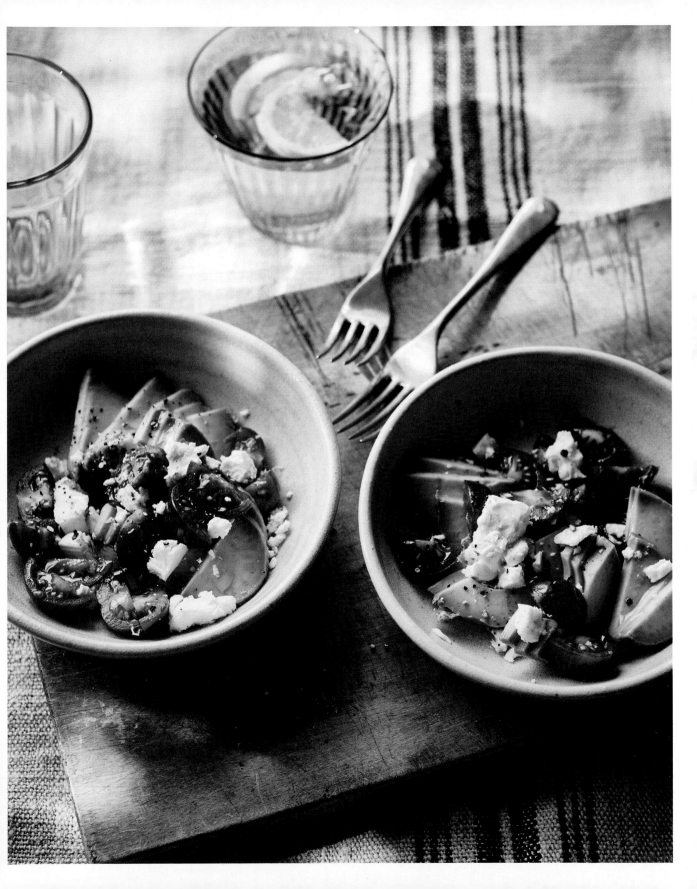

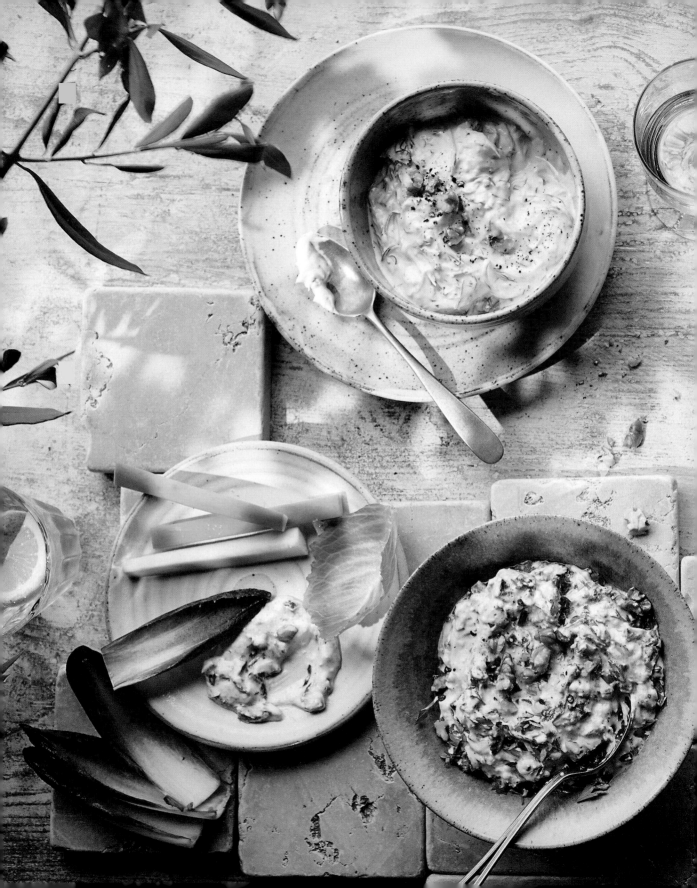

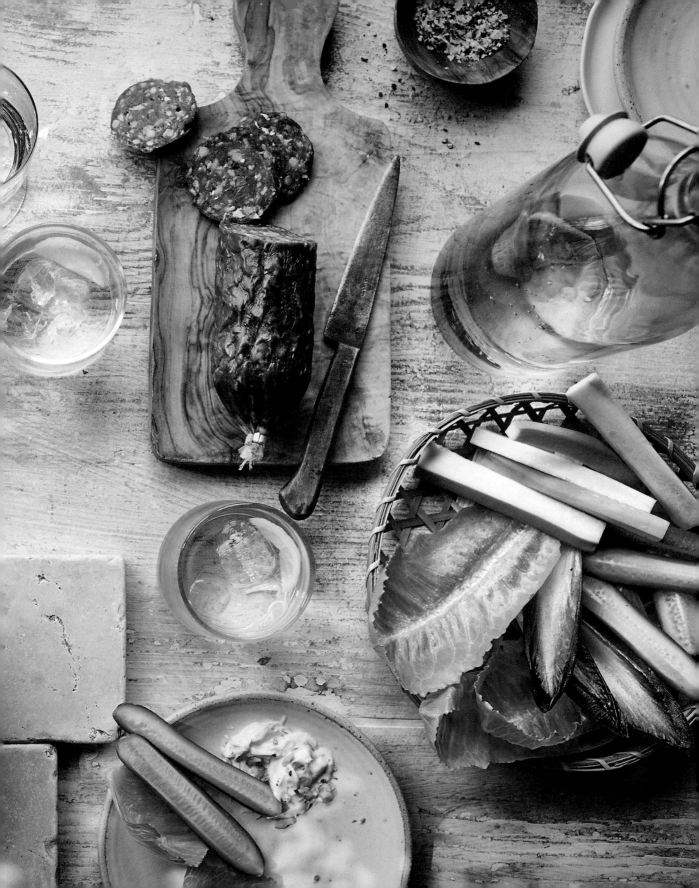

Bulgarian Meze

I was amazed by the delicious array of starter dishes known as мезе on our visit to Bulgaria. I could have included all of them but have chosen my two favourites. Both are made with strained live yogurt, which is thick and creamy. Also known as labneh, it is available in most supermarkets, or you can use Greek yogurt instead. Serve firm lettuce leaves, celery sticks, raw fennel or chicory to scoop up the dips. Add pickles, tomatoes, cold cuts or the Flatbreads from page 152. In Bulgaria it is served with the local rakiya, similar to grappa.

Katuk

SERVES 4

100g (3½oz) feta cheese

200g (7oz) thick, strained, full-fat yogurt

2 garlic cloves, grated (optional)

150g (5½oz) roast red peppers from a jar (drained weight), finely chopped

1–2 tablespoons unrefined sunflower or extra virgin olive oil

a small handful of flat-leaf parsley, stems and leaves finely chopped

50g (1¾oz) walnuts, finely chopped (optional)

salt and plenty of freshly ground black pepper

Per serving 6.5g net carbs, 0.9g fibre, 10g protein, 19.4g fat, 240kcal

Katuk is a cheese and red pepper paste served as an appetizer in Bulgaria. We were shown how to make this by our friend Srebrina Timofei who forms it into balls (with an ice-cream scoop). It is often decorated with walnuts and parsley. Since our trip to Bulgaria, I keep a jar of roast red peppers in the fridge or I make my own (see page 21); they provide instant flavour and I use them in omelettes, salads and in the Shopski Cheese on page 126. If you don't have them, add paprika or smoked paprika to taste instead. Traditionally Bulgarians use sunflower oil which we would only recommend if you can find an unrefined version, otherwise use olive oil. Black pepper is my own twist and isn't traditional.

Crumble the feta into a bowl or mash it roughly with a fork. Stir in the yogurt, garlic, if using, and lots of black pepper followed by the red peppers. Loosen the mixture with oil if it is very stiff – you need to be able to scoop it up with vegetables. Taste and add a little salt if necessary.

Transfer to a dish (or make the balls with an ice-cream scoop if you prefer) and scatter over the parsley and walnuts.

Snow White Salad

SERVES 4

3 heaped tablespoons thick, strained,
 full-fat yogurt

I long cucumber, peeled and
 coarsely grated

I teaspoon unrefined sunflower oil or
 extra virgin olive oil

I heaped tablespoon finely chopped
 dill leaves and stems

I small garlic clove, grated or crushed

salt, to taste

To serve

20g (¾oz) walnuts, crushed

freshly ground black pepper (optional)

Per serving 2.2g net carbs, 0.9g fibre,
2.4g protein, 5.4g fat, 66kcal

I was shown how to make this in Bulgaria by our friend Svetlana Nikolova. She used a mandolin and in seconds the cucumber was cut, but at home I use a coarse grater which works just as well. Svetlana showed me that if you add an equal amount of water to the salad, then you get the delicious tarator, a cold soup that is really popular on hot summer days.

First judge your yogurt. Most Bulgarians use thick, strained yogurt to make this fairly firm dip, however if your yogurt is less than firm, then it is better to squeeze some of the juice out of the cucumber after grating it.

Mix all the ingredients together in a bowl and season to taste. Scatter over the walnuts to serve and garnish with a twist of black pepper, if using.

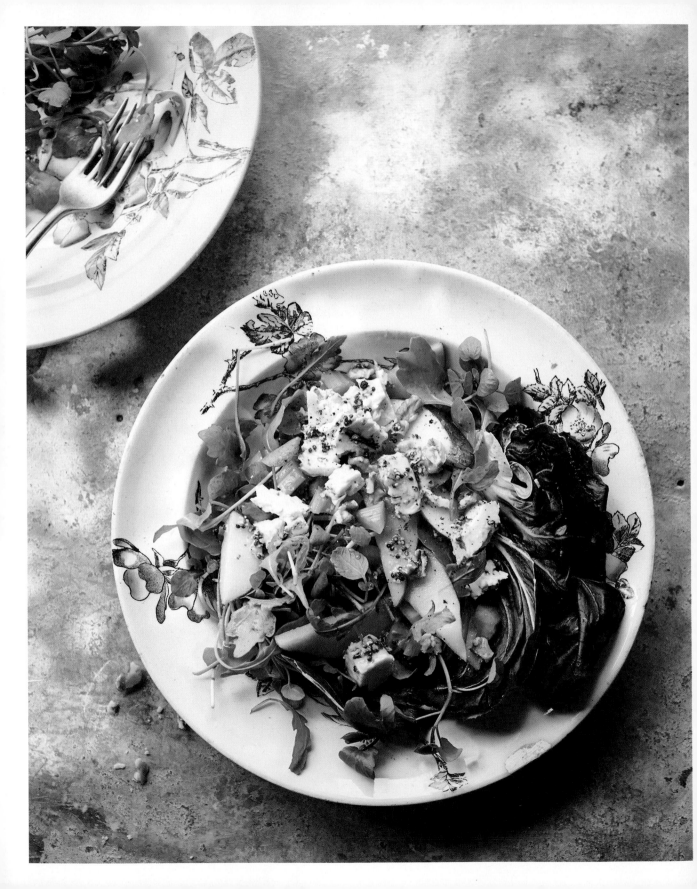

Blue Cheese, Pear & Watercress

SERVES 2

2 handfuls of watercress, rocket, chicory,
 radicchio or shredded cabbage

3 celery sticks, plus any leaves,
 roughly chopped

1 medium pear, cut into small cubes
 or sliced

40g (1½oz) walnuts, roughly chopped

100g (3½oz) blue cheese, such
 as Stilton, Gorgonzola Dolce
 or Roquefort

For the mustard dressing

1 teaspoon cider vinegar

3 tablespoons walnut or olive oil

1 teaspoon wholegrain or Dijon mustard

salt and freshly ground black pepper

Per serving 13g net carbs, 7g fibre,
17g protein, 48g fat, 560kcal

This recipe is lovely for a quick lunch. It is also good with the low-carb bread (page 110) or the Flaxseed Oatcakes on page 202. For colour, crunch and extra vitamins, I've suggested peppery watercress, but really any salad leaves or some finely shredded cabbage will do. Depending on the texture, crumble your blue cheese or slice it thinly.

Roughly tear the salad leaves and lay in the bottom of 2 bowls.

Mix all the dressing ingredients together in a mixing bowl and season to taste. Add the celery, pear and walnuts to the dressing and toss through. Divide between the 2 serving bowls, add the cheese and a twist of pepper and serve straight away.

Goat's Cheese, Black Onion Seed & Tomato Salad

SERVES 1

1 teaspoon black onion (nigella) seeds

50g (1¾oz) goat's cheese

4 cherry tomatoes, halved or quartered if large

1 medium beetroot, weighing about 75g (2½oz)

1 tablespoon extra virgin olive oil, plus extra for drizzling

1 teaspoon balsamic vinegar

a small handful of flat-leaf parsley, coriander or basil, roughly torn

salt and freshly ground black pepper

Per serving 9.6g net carbs, 4.4g fibre, 12.4g protein, 9.2g fat, 331kcal

I love the contrasts in this salad; dramatic black onion seeds strewn across crumbly white goat's cheese while the beetroot's blood-red juices mingle with the tomatoes and sweet balsamic vinegar. The idea came to me in a hurry when I had just 10 minutes to get a cheese-based supper ready for my first Zoom cheese and wine party. I spent so long on the new technology I ran out of time, but luckily this salad paired perfectly with an open bottle of fruity Roero Arneis.

Crush the black onion seeds in a pestle and mortar or scatter them on a board and roll over them with a wine bottle.

Put the cheese in a bowl and scatter over the crushed seeds. Chop the tomatoes and beetroot into the bowl, pour over the oil and balsamic vinegar and season with salt. Give everything a good twist of black pepper and one more drizzle of olive oil. Scatter over the herbs and serve straight away.

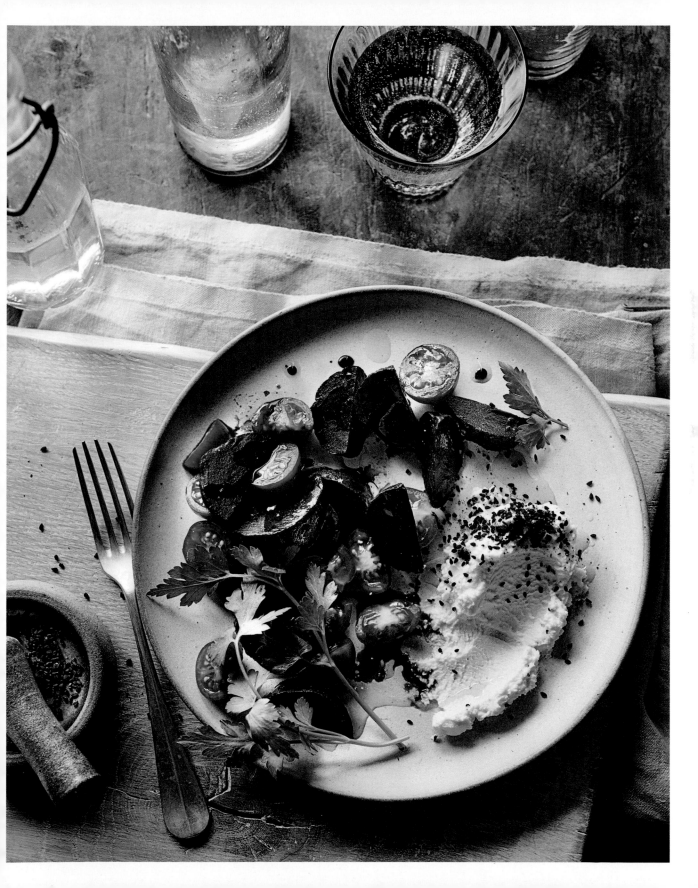

Lentil & Avocado Salad

SERVES 2

400g (14oz) can green lentils, drained

1 avocado, cubed

zest and juice of ½ lemon

15g (½oz) flat-leaf parsley, finely chopped

3 tablespoons extra virgin olive oil

salt and freshly ground black pepper

Per serving 30.8g net carbs, 16.7g fibre, 19.7g protein, 31.6g fat, 530kcal

A super-quick standby breakfast or lunch invented to appease the hunger of a teenager; it has been with us ever since. We also eat it as a side dish between four to cut the carbs and add to it in the form of cooked cold meat, roast peppers (see page 21) and fried or boiled eggs.

Mix all the ingredients together in a bowl and season to taste. Transfer to 2 serving dishes and enjoy.

Shopska Salad

SERVES 2

1 small red onion, finely sliced

½ long cucumber, cubed

2 roast red peppers from a jar
(75g/2½oz) or 1 red pepper,
cut into bite-sized pieces

1 green pepper, cut into
bite-sized pieces

2 large ripe tomatoes, top cores
removed and roughly chopped

10 Kalamata olives, stoned

2 tablespoons extra virgin olive oil

1 tablespoon red wine vinegar

a small bunch of flat-leaf parsley,
leaves roughly chopped, stalks
finely chopped

200g (7oz) feta cheese or Bulgarian
sirene (if you can find it)

salt and freshly ground black pepper

Per serving 15.9g net carbs, 5.5g
fibre, 17.3g protein, 38g fat, 482kcal

Our last trip abroad was to Sofia and Plovdiv in Bulgaria. I was really impressed by their range of meze; salads that were a happy blend of fresh and pickled vegetables, sirene (similar to feta) cheese, thick Bulgarian yogurt and plenty of fresh herbs. Bulgarian cooking is influenced by centuries of living under the Ottoman empire. The Russians freed them from the Turks after World War II, and they too had an impact on the food by standardizing and promoting certain dishes for tourists, such as this Shopska Salad. It has become the Bulgarian national dish as it combines the colours of their flag. The recipe uses fresh or roasted peppers, or you can use the Spanish ones sold in jars at most supermarkets. Find a brand you like or make your own (see page 21) and keep a jar in the fridge to make this dish, the Katuk on page 62 or the Shopski Cheese on page 126. Traditionally sunflower oil is used, but we prefer our best extra virgin olive oil.

Combine all the ingredients, apart from the cheese, in a mixing bowl and season to taste.

Divide between 2 bowls and coarsely grate the cheese over the top. Serve straight away or leave in the fridge for up to an hour.

New Russian Salad

SERVES 4

400g (14oz) mixture of carrots,
    cauliflower, radishes, crisp lettuce
    or chicory

25g (1oz) frozen peas

2 spring onions, finely sliced

150g (5½oz) cooked beetroot, cut
    into fingers

50g (1¾oz) gherkins, halved

a small bunch of dill fronds and stems
    or a few chives, finely chopped

For the horseradish mayo

3 tablespoons mayonnaise

3 tablespoons Greek yogurt

1 tablespoon lemon juice or
    cider vinegar

1 tablespoon horseradish sauce

1 teaspoon Dijon mustard

salt and freshly ground black pepper

Per serving 10.7g net carbs, 3.9g
fibre, 3.1g protein, 10g fat, 155kcal

This recipe simplifies Russian salad to allow all the ingredients to shine and omits the carby potatoes. The piquant creamy sauce marries well with smoked foods, such as salmon, mackerel or sausages. Try it with eggs or make it vegan with vegan mayo and chickpeas for protein. Use a mixture of vegetables to make up the bulk of the salad and if you do use dill, don't forget to include the stems; they are deliciously aniseedy.

Peel the carrots (if they need it) and cut them lengthways into quarters if small or if large, into matchsticks. Slice the cauliflower into bite-size pieces as thinly as you dare without the slices falling apart. Put the carrots, cauliflower and peas into a bowl and pour over half a kettle of boiling water and leave it to stand for 10 minutes.

Put the spring onions into a bowl of cold water to dilute their strength. Slice the radishes and separate the leaves of lettuce or chicory, if using.

Put the horseradish mayo ingredients in a small bowl and mix together. Taste and adjust the flavour accordingly; it should be punchy with heat from the horseradish and mustard.

Drain the carrots, cauliflower, peas and the spring onions. Neatly arrange or randomly throw on to a serving plate or wooden board, along with the beetroot, gherkins and remaining ingredients. Splash over the dressing and scatter the herbs over the top. Serve straight away or leave for up to 30 minutes at room temperature.

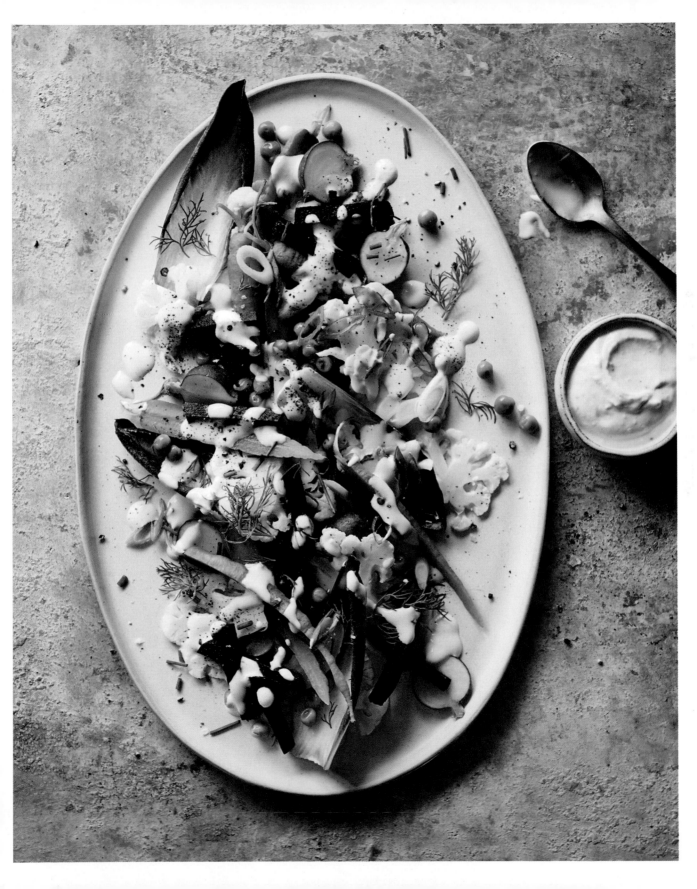

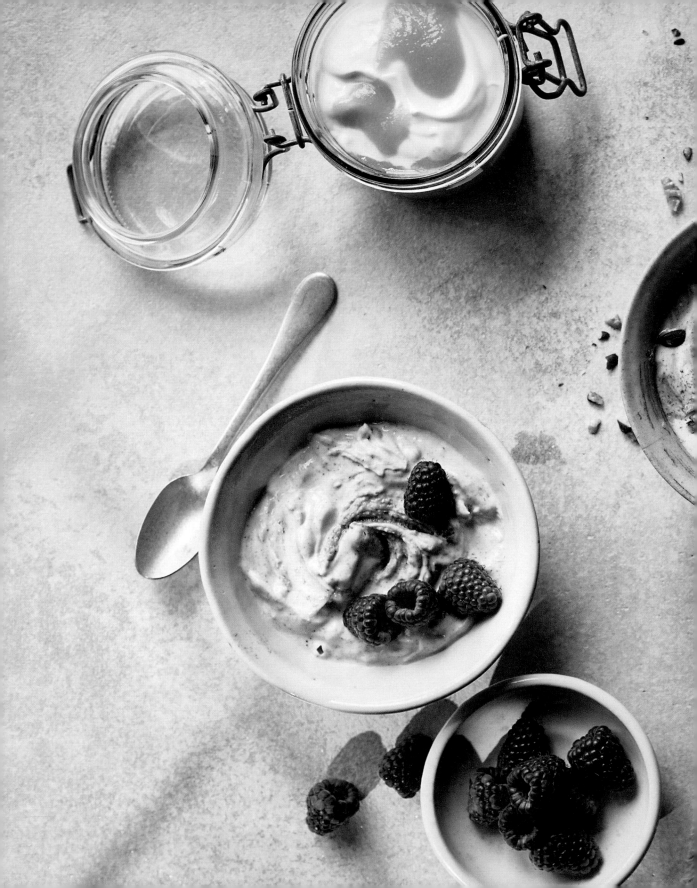

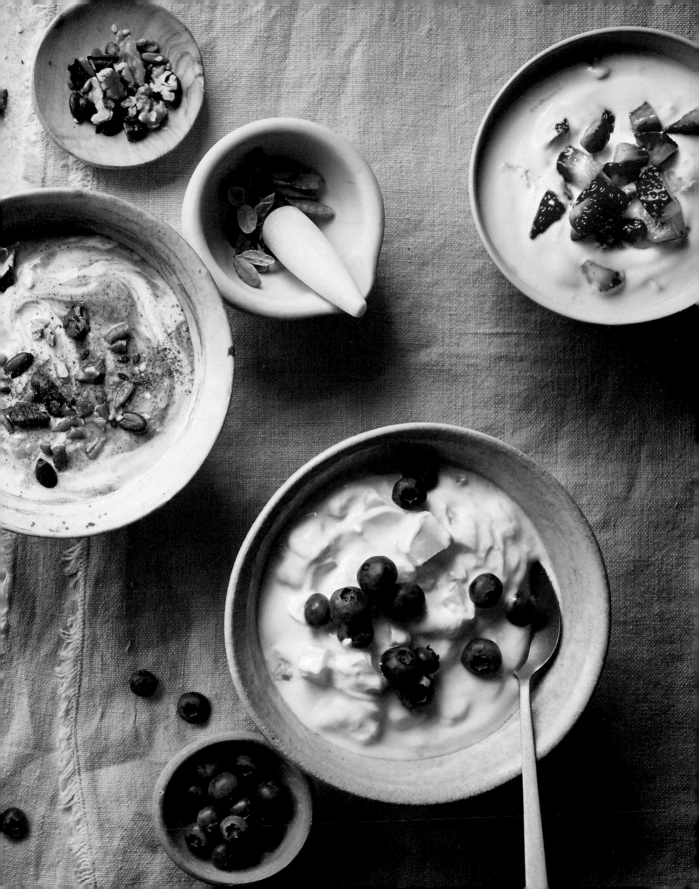

If all you can manage in the morning is emptying a punnet of raspberries over your yogurt, then go ahead, it will still be delicious and so much better than cereal. One step further is to mash the berries into the yogurt with a fork to release the flavour and a capful of vanilla extract stirred through makes it a treat. However, if you need a change, try one of the ideas here. You can always make it the night before and leave it in the fridge. Alternatively divide into four small servings and enjoy for dessert. Only add the honey if you need to. It will still be a lot less sugar than in commercial brands of fruity yogurt, which can contain up to 20g carbs per 150g (5½oz) serving without any additional fruit. Serve straight away or chill in the fridge until you want to eat.

Pear, Ginger & Blueberry Yogurt

SERVES 2

1 medium pear, peeled and diced

300g (10½oz) whole Greek yogurt

2 teaspoons vanilla extract

1 heaped tablespoon freshly
    grated ginger

1 teaspoon honey (optional)

100g (3½oz) blueberries

Per serving 23g net carbs, 3g fibre,
15g protein, 11g fat, 255kcal

Use fresh or canned pears for this recipe but do drain the canned juice away as it is usually full of sugar. You may need more ginger depending on the freshness of your root, so taste and adjust as necessary. I like it spicy, so I'm inclined to overdo it according to the rest of my family! Reduce the net carbs by 3g by leaving out the honey if you are strict low carb (see the CarbScale on page 29).

Stir all the ingredients, apart from the blueberries, together in a small mixing bowl. Divide between 2 glasses and top with the berries.

Chai Yogurt with Coconut

SERVES 2

4 cardamom pods, split, or
   ¼ teaspoon ground cardamom

100g (3½oz) coconut cream, top only

200g (7oz) whole Greek yogurt

2 teaspoons honey (optional)

1 teaspoon ground turmeric

2 teaspoons vanilla extract

1 teaspoon ground cinnamon, plus extra
   to garnish

2 tablespoon nuts, such as walnuts or
   pecans, roughly chopped

1 tablespoon seeds, such as sunflower,
   pumpkin, sesame or flax

Per serving 12.9g net carbs, 2.6g
fibre, 9.2g protein, 27g fat, 341kcal

We love the flavours of chai tea, so have combined them in a yogurt. It works really well as a fancy breakfast or as a dessert. Do use all coconut yogurt if you prefer. I find it quite strong, so use cow's milk yogurt and coconut cream, which is sold separately, or you can use the chilled and separated top of a can of coconut milk. Stir the remaining coconut milk into hot coffee or use in Charlotte's Dahl on page 141 or the Berry Smoothie on page 77.

If you are not using ground cardamom, split the cardamom pods open and crush the seeds with a pestle and mortar (chop them if you don't have one).

Stir all the ingredients, apart from the nuts and seeds, together in a small mixing bowl. Divide between 2 glasses and top with the nuts, seeds and a pinch more cinnamon.

Strawberry & Lemon Yogurt

SERVES 2

2 teaspoons vanilla extract, to taste

300g (10½oz) whole Greek yogurt

finely grated zest of ½ lemon

1 teaspoon honey (optional)

100g (3½oz) strawberries, roughly
   chopped, or other low-carb berry
   such as raspberries or blackberries,
   or a mixture

Per serving 12.7g net carbs, 1.4g
fibre, 6.5g protein, 9.3g fat, 173kcal

This is so simple to put together but tastes delicious. We love it as it is, especially if the strawberries are ripe and sweet, but if you have tart berries add a teaspoon of honey to the yogurt.

Stir the vanilla into the yogurt with the lemon zest and honey, if using. Taste and adjust as necessary with more lemon or vanilla.

Divide the mixture between 2 glasses and top with the berries.

Peanut Butter & Jelly Yogurt

SERVES 2

150g (5½oz) whole Greek yogurt

2 tablespoons smooth or crunchy peanut butter

1 teaspoon honey (optional)

2 teaspoons vanilla extract

50g (1¾oz) raspberries

Per serving 19.4g net carbs, 4.9g fibre, 12.9g protein, 24g fat, 376kcal

If you like the combination of peanut butter and jelly, you will love this. I have allowed pretty small portions as it is filling, so think of this as a small dessert rather than a meal.

Mix a little of the yogurt with the peanut butter and the honey, if using, together with a fork in a small bowl. Then stir in the remaining yogurt and the vanilla.

Spoon the peanut yogurt into 2 glasses and top with the raspberries.

Apricot Yogurt

SERVES 2

1 can apricots (235g/8½oz drained weight) or 235g (8½oz) fresh apricots

2 teaspoons honey

300g (10½oz) whole Greek yogurt

1 teaspoon vanilla extract

Per serving 20.3g net carbs, 2.3g fibre, 7g protein, 9.4g fat, 204kcal

Do use fresh apricots, nectarine or peaches when they are in season and ripe and flavourful. The rest of the year, a can of fruit, drained well, does the trick. Most of the sugar in canned fruit is in the juice, so do discard it.

Purée the apricots and honey together in a small food processor.

Mix the yogurt with the vanilla.

Divide half the purée between the bottom of 2 glasses. Top with the yogurt and finish with the remaining purée.

Berry Smoothie

SERVES 2

200g (7oz) frozen berries such as blueberries, raspberries, strawberries

400ml (14fl oz) full-fat coconut milk

2 teaspoons vanilla extract

Per serving 14.5g net carbs, 3.5g fibre, 3.4g protein, 30.2g fat, 384cal

This is our son Flavio's breakfast on the go; it's easy to make and drink and fills him up until lunchtime. He makes it in a high-speed blender and pours it into a cup with a lid, then sips it on the way to work. It's dairy free – which is great for him, but you can use cow's milk if you prefer or other plant-based milk.

Whizz the ingredients together in a high-speed blender until just smooth. Serve straight away.

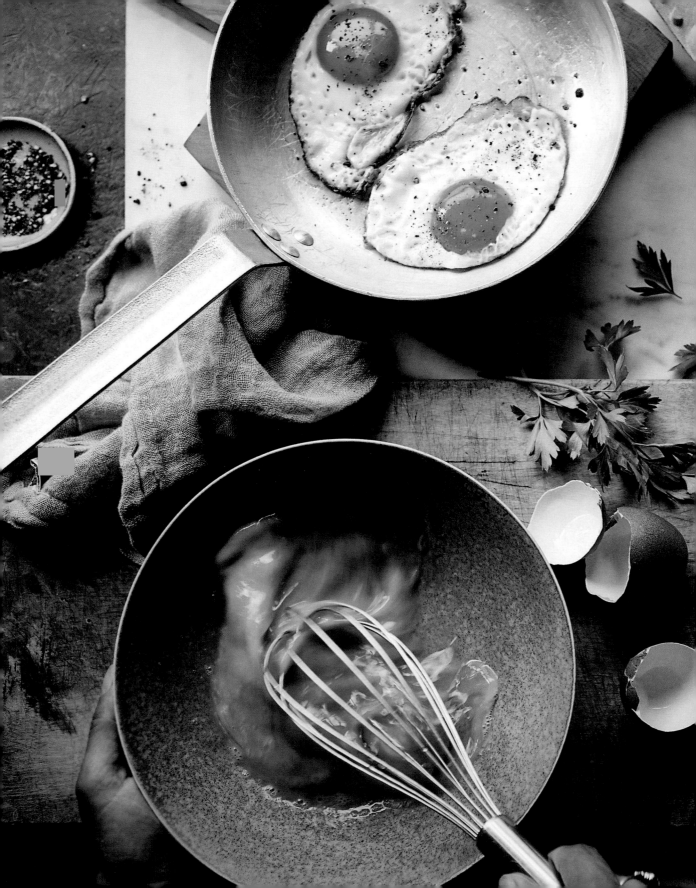

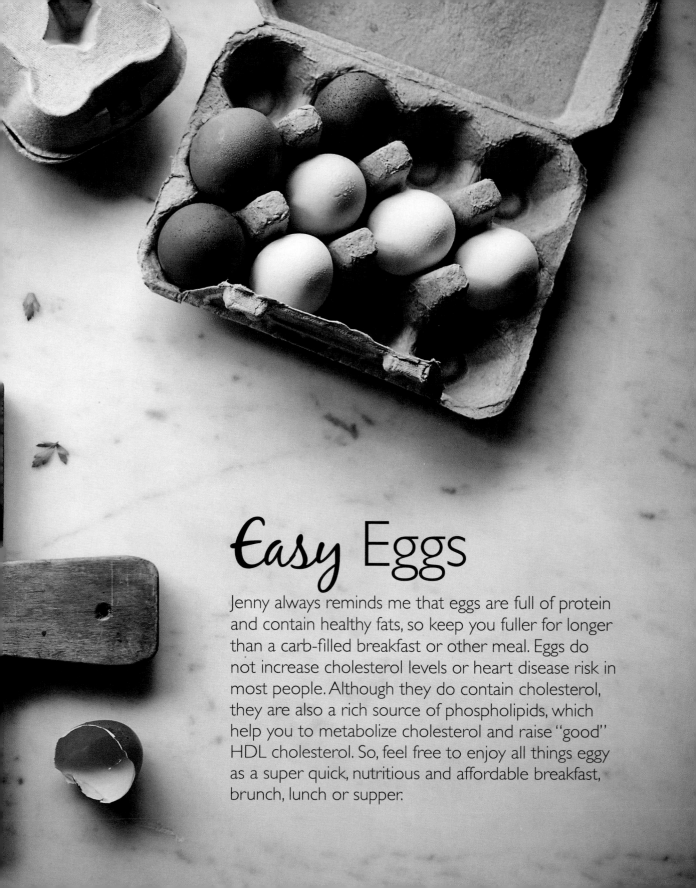

Easy Eggs

Jenny always reminds me that eggs are full of protein and contain healthy fats, so keep you fuller for longer than a carb-filled breakfast or other meal. Eggs do not increase cholesterol levels or heart disease risk in most people. Although they do contain cholesterol, they are also a rich source of phospholipids, which help you to metabolize cholesterol and raise "good" HDL cholesterol. So, feel free to enjoy all things eggy as a super quick, nutritious and affordable breakfast, brunch, lunch or supper.

The Spicy Green Omelette

SERVES 1

2 eggs

2 tablespoons coriander or flat-leaf
  parsley, leaves and stems,
  finely chopped

2 tablespoons double cream

1 hot red or green Thai chilli, finely sliced

a knob of butter

25g (1oz) mature Cheddar cheese,
  grated

a large handful of watercress and/or
  baby spinach, roughly chopped

salt and freshly ground black pepper

Per serving 2.4g net carbs, 0.2g fibre,
13.4g protein, 36g fat, 388kcal

This very quick and simple egg recipe has become known as the green omelette in our house. The point was to get our teenagers to eat super-nutritious greens on something that could be prepared quickly when hunger drove them out of their bedrooms! The topping choices are infinite and depend on what's in the fridge. If the chilli is very hot, add a dollop of thick yogurt. We love tomatoes, so often serve a couple on the side for colour.

Make sure you have a warm plate ready and everything you need to hand to work quickly.

Crack the eggs into a bowl and add the coriander, cream and chilli and whisk with a fork until well combined. Season with plenty of black pepper and a pinch of salt. Set aside.

Melt the butter in a non-stick frying pan over a medium heat. Swirl it around to coat the base of the pan. Increase the heat to high and add the eggs. Use a spatula to move the eggs around for about a minute, criss-crossing the pan to get the runny eggs to the bottom but making sure there are no holes in the omelette. When the outer edges become opaque, run the spatula around the rim of the pan to loosen it. Shake the pan to make sure the omelette can slide.

Scatter cheese over the whole omelette followed by the watercress. Reeuce the heat to low, put on the lid and leave for couple of minutes. Serve straight away.

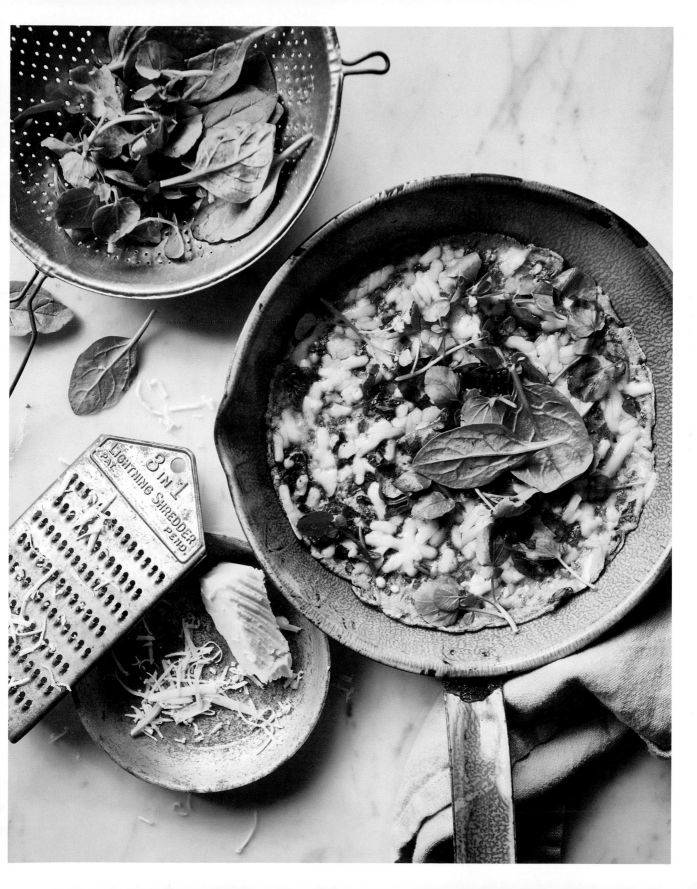

The Stuffed Omelette with Goat's Cheese & Spinach

SERVES 1

2 eggs

2 tablespoons double cream

a knob of butter

1 heaped tablespoon crumbly cheese, such as goat's cheese or feta or grated Cheddar

1 heaped tablespoon cream cheese, crème fraîche or thick Greek yogurt

30g (1oz) baby spinach or watercress, roughly chopped

1 heaped tablespoon finely chopped fresh herbs, such as chives, flat-leaf parsley or tarragon

salt and freshly ground black pepper

Per serving 2.3g net carbs, 0.3g fibre, 11.1g protein, 38g fat, 397kcal

I wanted to call this *omelette aux fine herbes* as it reminds me of my 1970s school cookery lessons where we had to master the art of the omelette. However, the "Frenchness" can conjure up something complicated and a stuffed omelette just isn't. In this case it is simply a combination of eggs and whatever cheese, green leaves and herbs you have. A mixture of green herbs gives the *fine herbes* flavour but just an omelette on its own is equally good. Further additions include leftover roast vegetables or cooked ham.

Make sure you have a warm plate ready and everything you need to hand to work quickly.

Crack the eggs into a bowl, add the cream, then whisk with a fork until well combined. Season with plenty of black pepper and a pinch of salt. Set aside.

Melt the butter in a non-stick frying pan over a medium heat. Swirl it around to coat the base of the pan. Increase the heat to high and add the eggs. Use a spatula to move the eggs around for about a minute, criss-crossing the pan to get the runny eggs to the bottom but making sure there are no holes in the omelette. When the outer edges become opaque, run the spatula around the rim of the pan to loosen it. Shake the pan to make sure the omelette can slide.

Cook for 2–3 minutes or until the eggs are just cooked. Crumble the cheese over half the omelette and use a teaspoon to dollop over the cream cheese. Then add the spinach and herbs and use a large spatula or slice to flip the uncovered side over to form a semicircle. Reduce the heat to low, put on the lid and leave for couple of minutes. Serve straight away.

The Cheese & Ham Omelette

SERVES 1

2 eggs

2 tablespoons double cream

a knob of butter

25g (1oz) mature Cheddar cheese, grated

25g (1oz) cooked ham, torn or diced

salt and freshly ground black pepper

Per serving 2.3g net carbs, 0g fibre, 21g protein, 38g fat, 439kcal

I had often overlooked the humble omelette as something too simple, too humdrum. That is until a guest at a hotel where we were staying requested one for breakfast and I ordered one too and realized quite how delicious they were. Why had I been ignoring them for 20 years? Welcome back to my life Cheese & Ham Omelette, and please stay a while. Any cheese will work, some crumble, some need to be grated and others can only be sliced – try them all or mix them up as you like. Any cooked ham, torn ham hock or bacon is good or leave it out if you prefer. I like this omelette with mustard on the side.

Make sure you have a warm plate ready and everything you need to hand to work quickly.

Crack the eggs into a bowl and add the cream, then whisk with a fork until well combined. Season with plenty of black pepper and a pinch of salt. Set aside.

Melt the butter in a non-stick frying pan over a medium heat. Swirl it around to coat the base of the pan. Increase the heat to high and add the eggs. Use a spatula to move the eggs around for about a minute, criss-crossing the pan to get the runny eggs to the bottom but making sure there are no holes in the omelette. When the outer edges become opaque, run the spatula around the rim of the pan to loosen it. Shake the pan to make sure the omelette can slide.

Cook for 2–3 minutes until the eggs are just cooked. Scatter the cheese and ham over half the omelette and use a large spatula or slice to flip the uncovered side over to form a semicircle. Reduce the heat to low, put on the lid and leave for couple of minutes. Serve straight away.

Mushroom Rarebit with Poached Eggs

SERVES 2

2 large portobello mushrooms, brushed clean and stalks cut away

2 teaspoons extra virgin olive oil

3 eggs

35g (1¼oz) mature Cheddar or other hard cheese, grated

½ teaspoon Dijon mustard

a couple of drops of Worcestershire sauce

1 heaped tablespoon Greek yogurt

salt and freshly ground black pepper

Per serving 3.8g net carbs, 2.8g fibre, 22g protein, 20g fat, 290kcal

This is an easy brunch or a light supper. Serve on its own, with sautéed spinach or a crisp, green salad (page 57) on the side.

Preheat the grill to high.

Lay the mushrooms cut-side up on a wire rack over a baking tray, brush with the oil and season with salt and pepper. Grill for 7 minutes or until tender and darker around the edges. Using tongs, turn the mushrooms over so the domed sides are facing upward and grill for 3 minutes.

Meanwhile, make the filling. Mix one of the eggs together with the remaining ingredients in a bowl using a fork or whisk. Fill a frying pan or saucepan with water and bring to the boil.

Remove the mushrooms from the oven and spoon the filling into their cavities. Grill for 5–7 minutes or until golden brown. Any extra filling can be cooked in a ramekin at the same time.

Reduce the heat under the pan of water to medium, and when the water is bubbling, gently crack one egg into a teacup. Put the teacup into the water and tip it up so that the egg gently floats out. Repeat with the second egg. This method allows you to poach several eggs at once, depending on the size of your pan. Cook for 3–5 minutes, depending on how you like your eggs. Remove with a slotted spoon allowing any water to fall away.

Top each mushroom with a poached egg and serve straight away.

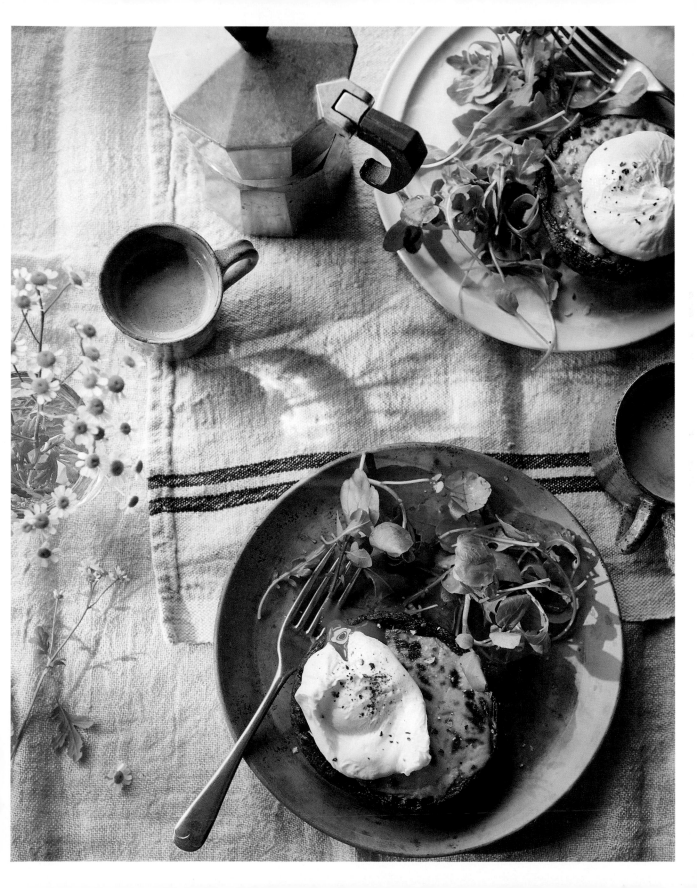

Quichata

SERVES 4

75g (2½oz) frozen peas

50g (1¾oz) butter

1 medium onion, finely chopped

100g (3½oz) streaky, smoked bacon, roughly chopped

5 eggs

150g (5½oz) ricotta cheese, soured cream or crème fraîche

50g (1¾oz) Parmesan or mature Cheddar cheese, grated

½ teaspoon salt and plenty of freshly ground black pepper

Per serving 9.1g net carbs, 1.3g fibre, 18g protein, 29.2g fat, 375kcal

Additions

200g (7oz) roast vegetables

120g (4¼oz) cooked ham, diced

200g (7oz) different cheeses, such as goat's cheese or feta

a large handful of chopped herbs, such as chives or thyme

2 x cans tuna, approx. 120g (4¼oz) drained weight

I wanted all the flavour of a traditional Quiche Lorraine in a frittata style that I could make in less than 30 minutes, so came up with the Quichata! This is a great basic recipe that can be adapted to use what's in your fridge and cupboards, or you can try some of the suggestions below. It's good hot or cold and perfect for lunchboxes. It also reheats well in a microwave.

Preheat the grill to high.

Plunge the peas into a bowl of just-boiled water for 5 minutes, then drain and set aside.

Melt half the butter in a medium non-stick, ovenproof frying pan. Add the onion and bacon and cook over a medium-high heat for 5 minutes or until the onion is soft.

Meanwhile, mix the eggs, ricotta, Parmesan and some seasoning together in a large mixing bowl. Add the peas and stir through. Tip the cooked bacon and onion into the mixture and stir through. Clean the pan with kitchen paper or give it a quick rinse and put back over a medium-high heat.

Melt the remaining butter and pour the egg mixture in. Cook for 5 minutes and then transfer to the grill for 8 minutes, near the hot surface, on a rack. When the quichata is set, remove from the oven with oven gloves. Be careful not to touch the handle (I have regretted this so many times!). Slide the quichata on to a warm serving plate or a wooden board and serve straight away or leave to cool to room temperature.

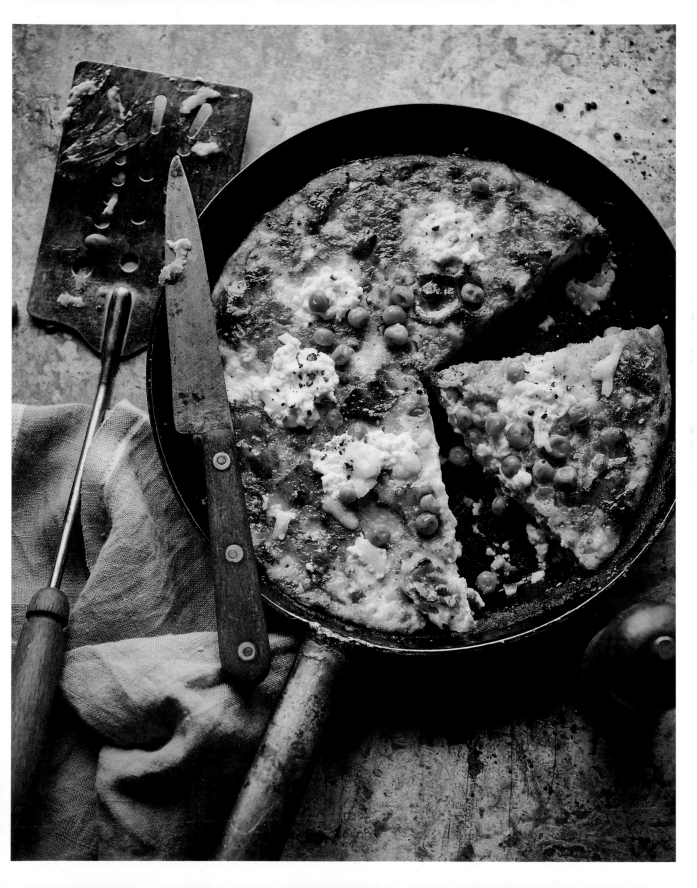

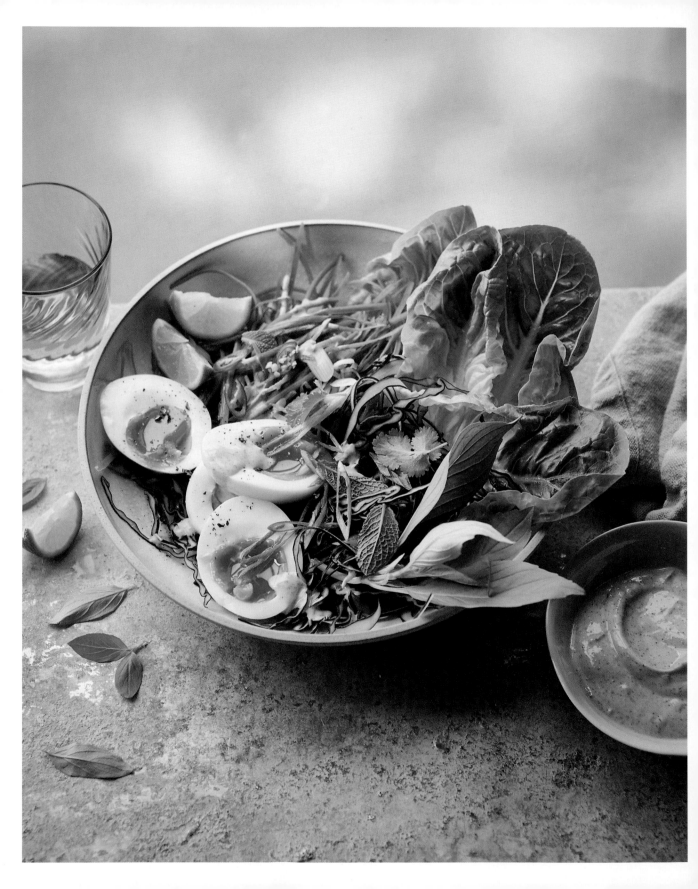

Boiled Eggs with Gado Gado

SERVES 4

8 eggs at room temperature

4 spring onions

a handful of salad leaves, such as
  Romaine or Little Gem

200g (7oz) red or white cabbage,
  finely shredded

2 medium carrot, scrubbed and grated

I hot Thai green chilli or jalapeño chilli
  from a jar, finely sliced

a large handful of one or a mixture of
  Thai basil, coriander and mint

2 tablespoons extra virgin olive oil

salt and freshly ground black pepper

For the dressing

I garlic clove, grated

2 tablespoons peanut butter

I hot Thai green or jalapeño chilli,
  finely sliced, or 1–2 teaspoons hot
  chilli powder

juice of 1–2 limes

100g (3½oz) Greek yogurt

3–4 teaspoons tamari or dark or light
  soy sauce

2 teaspoons fish sauce (optional)

Per serving 7.6g net carbs, 2g fibre,
10.6g protein, 16g fat, 222kcal

I always have cabbage in the fridge as it lasts a long time. Do add other raw vegetables to change the salad, such as grated swede, parsnip or turnip. Grated apple adds a touch of natural sweetness too. If you don't eat eggs, replace them with toasted nuts.

Fill a saucepan with water, bring to the boil and cook the eggs for 7 minutes for soft-boiled.

Finely slice the spring onions on the diagonal and put in a bowl of cold water for a few minutes to dilute their strength.

Lay the lettuce leaves into 4 bowls in piles. Make the dressing by mixing the ingredients together in a bowl, adding the lime juice and tamari to taste.

Drain the spring onions, then mix with the remaining ingredients in a bowl and season to taste. Cut the eggs open and lay over the salad with the dressing on the side. Any leftover lime can be squeezed over the dish.

Kale Stir-fry & Fried Eggs Over Easy

SERVES 4

2 tablespoons extra virgin olive oil

1 onion, finely chopped

1 red pepper, finely sliced

2 garlic cloves, finely sliced

a little finely chopped hot red or
  green chilli or a pinch of chilli flakes

10 cherry tomatoes, halved or
  quartered

400g (14oz) kale, cavolo nero or other
  cabbage, shredded

2 tablespoons ghee, lard or dripping

4 eggs

salt and freshly ground black pepper

Per serving 5.3g net carbs, 2g fibre,
6.5g protein, 14.7g fat, 184kcal

Dark leafy vegetables are so good for you as they are full of antioxidants and folate. Kale is a terrific source of vitamin K for healthy bones and teeth. If you don't eat eggs, stir in some cooked, drained beans for protein or enjoy this with sausages, meat or chicken. The best fats to fry the eggs in are ghee, lard or dripping. Coconut oil is also good, but I wouldn't mix its tropical flavour with this Mediterranean-style recipe.

Heat the oil in a large frying pan. Add the onion, red pepper, garlic, chilli (to taste) and some seasoning and fry over a medium heat for about 5 minutes, then add the tomatoes and cook for 2 minutes or until softened.

Meanwhile, boil or steam the kale for about 5 minutes until soft. Drain and add to the pan. Toss through, then taste and season as necessary.

To fry the eggs, add the fat to a frying pan over a medium-high heat. When it feels hot to your hand held above it, crack the eggs into the pan, socially distanced apart if your pan allows it. Season the eggs with a little salt and pepper. Fry for a couple of minutes or until you can see the white is mainly opaque and the yolk is starting to set. Remove them from the pan if you like them runny. If not, leave for longer or flip over with a spatula and leave for 30 seconds. This will give you eggs over easy, meaning the whites are cooked through and just the centres of the yolks are runny – just how I like them.

Serve the kale stir-fry in warm bowls topped with the fried eggs.

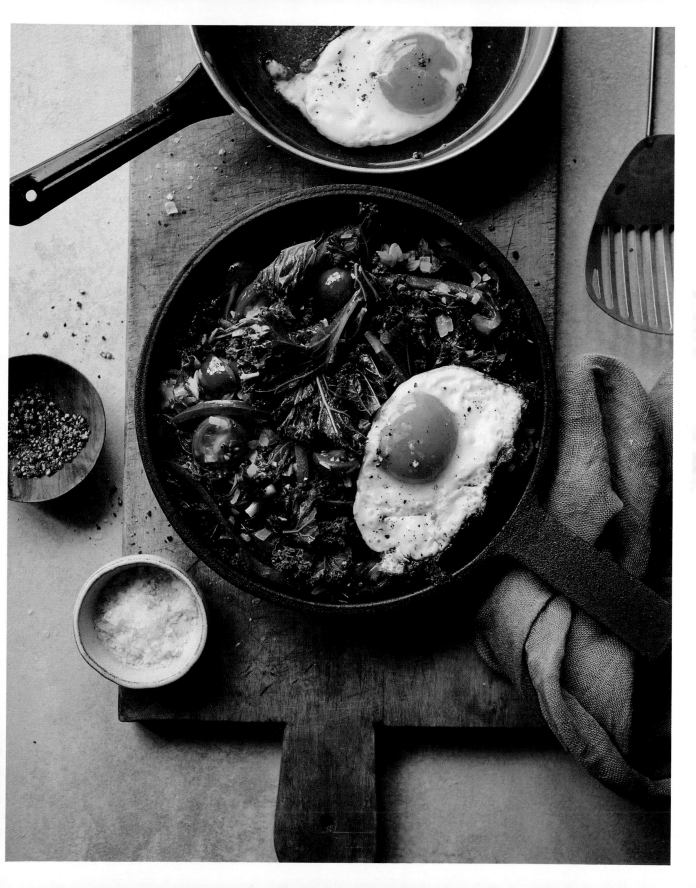

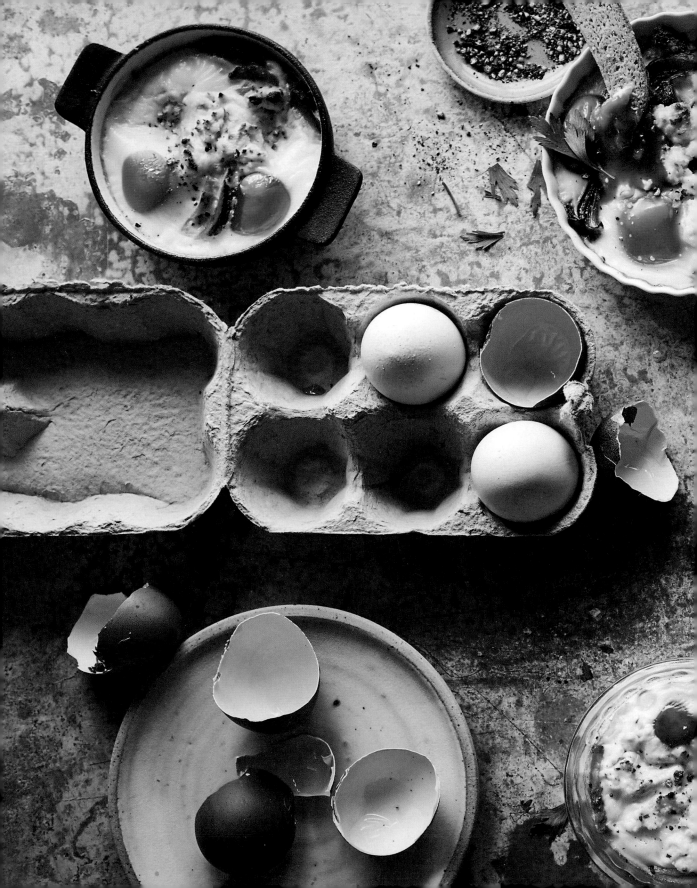

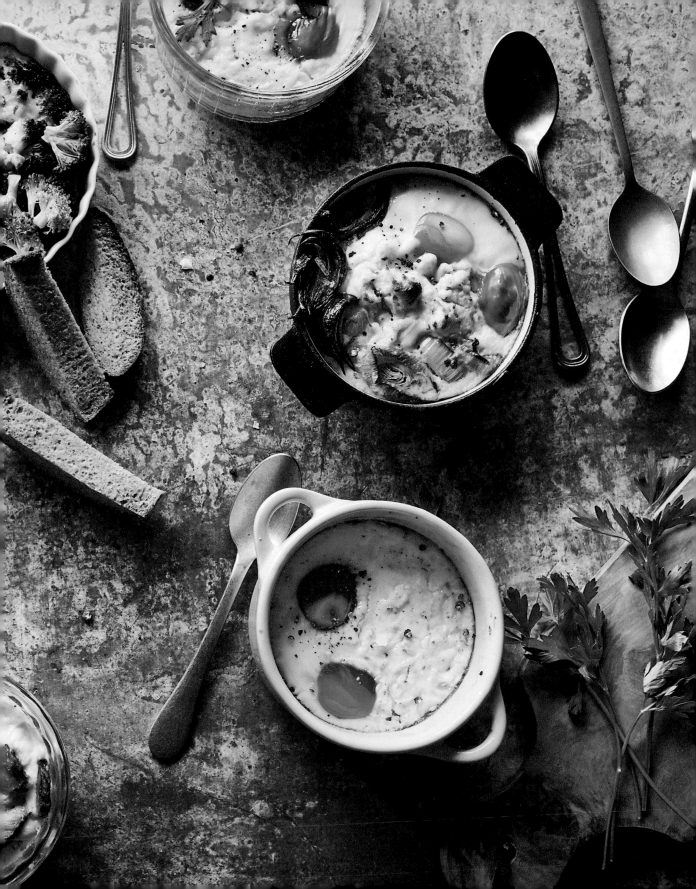

Boursin Baked Eggs

SERVES 2

2 teaspoons butter, softened,
  for greasing

4 eggs

2 heaped tablespoons Boursin or
  other grated cheese, such as Gruyère
  or Parmesan

2 tablespoons finely chopped herbs,
  such as tarragon, flat-leaf parsley or
  basil (optional)

4 tablespoons double cream

salt and freshly ground black pepper
  (unless you use Boursin)

Per serving 1g net carbs, 0.5g fibre,
16g protein, 40g fat, 430kcal

Our boys have a bit of a thing for Boursin, the creamy crumbly cheese that comes in different flavours, as it provides instant tang whenever they need something savoury. If you don't have it, use any cheese and herbs you do have to make these little pots of eggy loveliness.

You can use up leftover roast vegetables, cooked ham or bacon by placing them at the bottom of the ramekins after buttering. Baked eggs are surprisingly filling but if you need them to be more substantial serve them with buttered Baps on page 110 cut into soldiers.

If you don't have ramekins, use any small ovenproof bowls or teacups large enough to fit 2 eggs. However, different materials conduct the heat in varying ways, so you might find some eggs are cooked faster than others. Buttering the dishes makes it easy to spoon the mixture out when eating and helps with washing up later!

Preheat the oven to 240°C/220°C fan/475°F/gas mark 9. Butter 2 ramekins with a brush or your finger.

Crack 2 eggs into each ramekin. Crumble over the Boursin or grated cheese. Scatter over the herbs, if using, and pour 2 tablespoons of cream over each ramekin. Season with a little salt and pepper if you aren't using the Boursin.

Bake for 8–10 minutes or until the egg whites are just set but the yolks are still runny. Leave for a couple of minutes before serving. They will continue cooking in the residual heat and will be very hot to eat!

Feta & Herb Mini Frittatas

MAKES 6 FRITTATAS

4 eggs

100g (3½oz) feta or 25g (1oz)
   Parmesan cheese, finely grated

50g (1¾oz) one or mixture of herbs,
   such as flat-leaf parsley and
   coriander, leaves roughly chopped
   and stems finely chopped

salt and freshly ground black pepper

Per serving 1.1g net carbs, 0.1g fibre,
6.3g protein, 6.7g fat, 91kcal

Whether you use wilted herbs found in the back of the fridge or foraged wild herbs, do try these little frittatas. You can use just one herb, such as parsley, or a mixture. Don't forget that stems of parsley and coriander should be chopped finely but do add them as they have so much flavour.

These frittatas are so easy to whip up and very versatile. Try adding different cheeses, such as soft Gorgonzola, Boursin or Cheddar. Add in leftover roast vegetables, cooked bacon or tuna for just some of the variations. Mini frittatas are great for lunchboxes, breakfast or parties. If you have leftover egg white, use the same weight as one egg.

Preheat the oven to 220°C/200°C fan/425°F/gas mark 7. Prepare 6 small muffin cases or grease a shallow muffin tin.

Whisk all the ingredients together in a bowl and pour into the cases. Bake for 15 minutes or until firm to the touch and cooked through. Remove from the oven and eat straight away or leave to cool to room temperature. The frittatas will keep in the fridge for up to 3 days.

Grilled Asparagus, Cheese & Eggs

SERVES 2

8 asparagus spears, woody
   stems removed

3 eggs

1 tablespoon double cream

a knob of butter

3 heaped tablespoons cream cheese
   or Boursin

20g (¾oz) Parmesan or Cheddar
   cheese, grated

salt and freshly ground black pepper

Per serving 4.2g net carbs, 1g fibre,
13.1g protein, 31.5g fat, 352kcal

This is a great way of making an omelette puff up like a pizza and it's the same method I used for the Pizza Omelette in *The Reverse Your Diabetes Cookbook*. I've used asparagus and cream cheese here, but you could use roast vegetables, red pepper, feta or halloumi cheese instead.

Preheat the grill to high.

Steam or boil the asparagus until tender. This will take 5–8 minutes depending on their width. Drain and set aside.

While the asparagus cooks, beat the eggs with the cream and some seasoning in a small bowl.

Heat an ovenproof, non-stick frying pan over a medium-high heat and add the butter. Increase the heat to high and when the butter starts to foam, add the eggs. Use a spatula to move the eggs around for about a minute, criss-crossing the pan to get the runny eggs to the bottom but making sure there are no holes in the omelette. When the outer edges become opaque, run the spatula around the rim of the pan to loosen it. Shake the pan to make sure the omelette can slide.

When the eggs are almost set on the base of the pan, remove it from the heat. Dollop on the cream cheese, lay over the asparagus and scatter over the Parmesan. Season with a little salt and pepper (unless you have used Boursin as it has enough seasoning).

Put the pan under the hot grill, quite close to the source of heat, for 3–5 minutes or until the cheese has melted and the edges have risen and browned. Remove the pan from the grill using oven gloves and slide the omelette on to the warm plate.

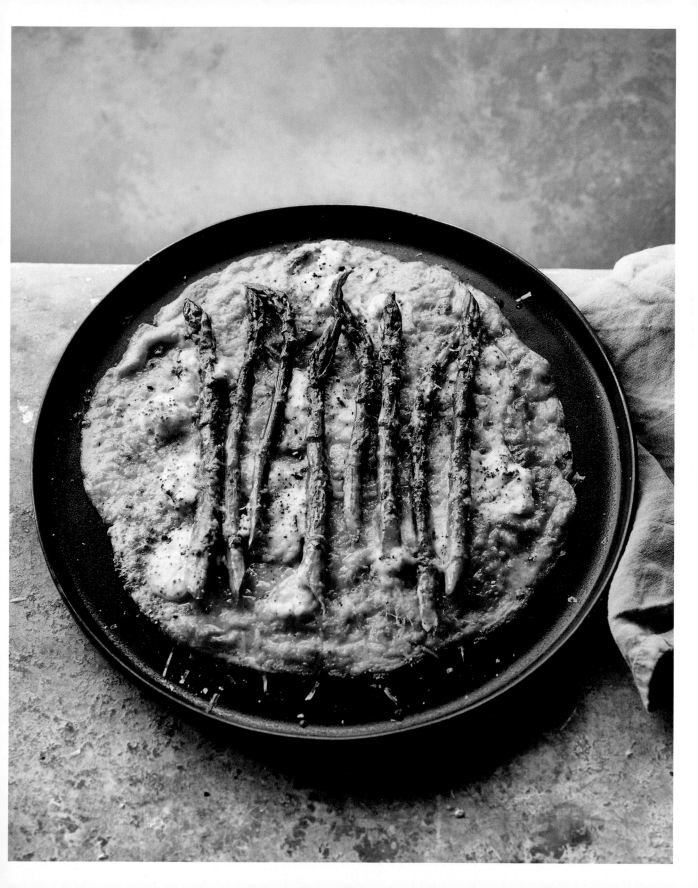

Simple Scrambled Eggs

SERVES 2

4 eggs

2 tablespoons double cream or
   crème fraîche

25g (1oz) butter, ghee, coconut or
   extra virgin olive oil

salt and freshly ground black pepper

Per serving 1.2g net carbs, 0g fibre,
11.6g protein, 24.8g fat, 276kcal

This is the basic recipe for creamy scrambled eggs. Enjoy on their own, or add a slice of smoked salmon, chopped fresh herbs, celery leaves, baby spinach, crumbled feta or halved cherry tomatoes.

Beat the eggs, cream, ½ teaspoon of salt and a few generous twists of black pepper together in a mixing bowl with a fork.

Melt the butter in a large, non-stick frying pan over a low heat until it starts to foam. Pour in the egg mixture and stir continuously as it begins to set. Move the runny eggs and solid areas together until it is cooked to your liking. Remove from the heat and serve straight away.

Mish Mash Misho-style

SERVES 2

2 tablespoons extra virgin olive oil

1 onion, finely chopped

1 large roast red pepper from a jar
   (approx. 100g/3½oz), roughly chopped

1 large tomato, diced

3 eggs

a small bunch of flat-leaf parsley, stems
   finely chopped and leaves roughly
   chopped

10g (¼oz) butter

100g (3½oz) feta cheese, crumbled

½ teaspoon paprika

¼ teaspoon ground fenugreek (optional)

Per serving 12.6g net carbs, 3.9g
fibre, 18.1g protein, 37.7g fat, 469kcal

I was introduced to Mish Mash in Bulgaria by our friend's son Misho; this egg, pepper and cheese delight is served in various ways in homes and restaurants across the country. It is personalized with garlic, peppers, other vegetables and fresh herbs but the important ingredient is the famous Bulgarian sharena or mixed salt. It is a blend of salt and dried ground herbs such as summer savoury, paprika, fenugreek, basil, thyme and others. You can find it online, but I find a pinch of fenugreek and paprika is equally delicious.

Heat the oil in a non-stick frying pan and fry the onion for 5 minutes or until just soft. Add the pepper and tomato and stir through to heat for a couple of minutes.

Crack the eggs into the pan and immediately stir them in. Keep stirring as they cook, add a little parsley and save a little for later. Add the butter on top in flecks and stir into the pan.

Next, add the feta and wait for it to soften a little before scattering over the spices. Stir through, then serve straight away scattered with the remaining parsley.

Hot & Spicy Scrambled Eggs

SERVES 2

¼ teaspoon mustard seeds

a knob of butter or ghee

1 small onion, finely sliced into half-moons

10 fresh or 15 dried curry leaves (optional)

a little hot green or red chilli, to taste, or ½ teaspoon chilli flakes

4 eggs

2 tablespoons double cream or crème fraîche

1 large tomato, diced

½ teaspoon ground turmeric

a small handful of coriander or flat-leaf parsley, stalks finely chopped and leaves roughly chopped

2 heaped tablespoons Greek yogurt

salt and freshly ground black pepper

Per serving 9g net carbs, 1.6g fibre, 13.7g protein, 26.5g fat, 327kcal

I love the flavour of fresh curry leaves and whenever I see them, I buy a bunch and keep them in the freezer. Find them in Asian shops and some large supermarkets. The dried leaves will do but they don't offer the same intensity of flavour. This is a perfect brunch or easy supper dish for two.

Put the mustard seeds in a non-stick frying pan over a medium-high heat and cook until they pop. Warm a couple of bowls.

Add the butter to the pan and when it foams add the onion, curry leaves and chilli. Season and continue to cook for about 8 minutes, stirring frequently.

Meanwhile, crack the eggs into a bowl and whisk with the cream and some seasoning.

Add the tomato and turmeric to the pan. Stir and cook for a couple of minutes, then pour in the eggs. Mix gently and cook for a couple of minutes, stirring continuously, until the eggs are done to your liking. Stir in the coriander and divide between the 2 warm bowls. Dollop on the yogurt and eat straight away.

Carbonara

SERVES 4

1 small leek, weighing about 175g (6oz),
  or 1 medium onion, finely chopped

150g (5½oz) smoked pancetta or
  streaky bacon, thinly sliced

2 tablespoons pork fat or olive oil

500g (1lb 2oz) cabbage, excluding stalk,
  cut into ribbons

75g (2½oz) frozen peas

25g (1oz) butter

100ml (3½fl oz) double cream

100g (3½oz) Pecorino Romano or
  Parmigiano Reggiano cheese, finely
  grated

4 eggs

salt and freshly ground black pepper

Per serving 15.5g net carbs, 4.5g
fibre, 22.7g protein, 44.8g fat, 558kcal

Carbonara is named after the *carbonari*, the charcoal makers around Rome who fed themselves on the cured meat, cheese and pasta they carried with them into the forest. Presumably specks of charcoal gave the dish extra flavour, although now they are replaced with black pepper. I have deconstructed an Italian classic – something I thought I would never admit to – in order to make this recipe equally delicious on ribbons of cabbage rather than strands of pasta.

Cook the leek and pancetta in the fat in a large frying pan over a medium heat until cooked through and slightly browned and crisp.

Put the cabbage and peas in a saucepan with a splash of water, the butter and some seasoning and cover with a lid. Cook for about 5 minutes or until soft. Drain thoroughly in a colander and add to the pan with the leek and bacon. Add the cream and cheese and stir through. Keep warm while you poach the eggs.

Poach the eggs following the method on page 84. Divide the creamy cabbage ribbons between 4 warm bowls and top each with an egg and a twist of black pepper; serve straight away.

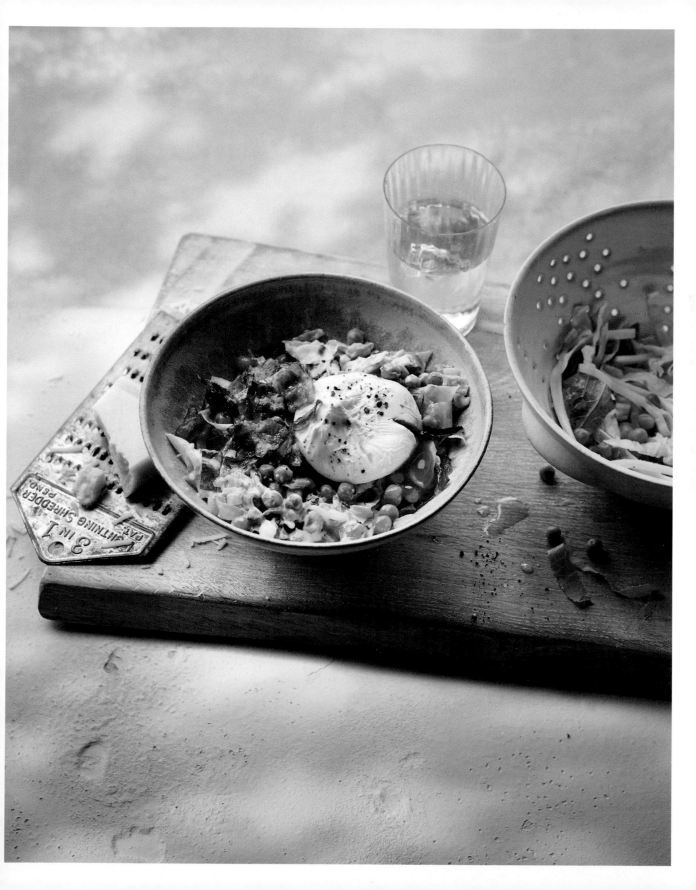

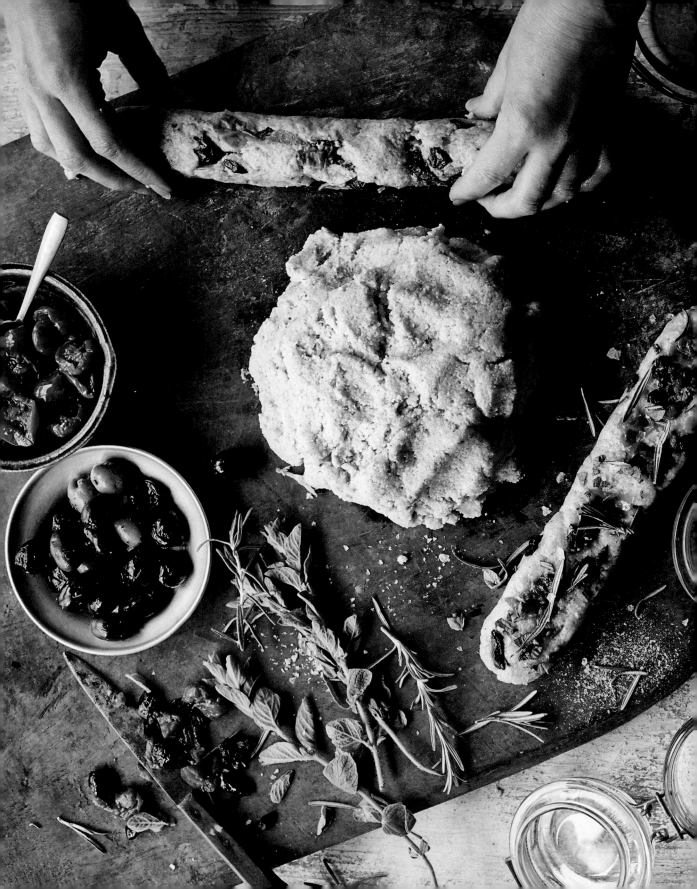

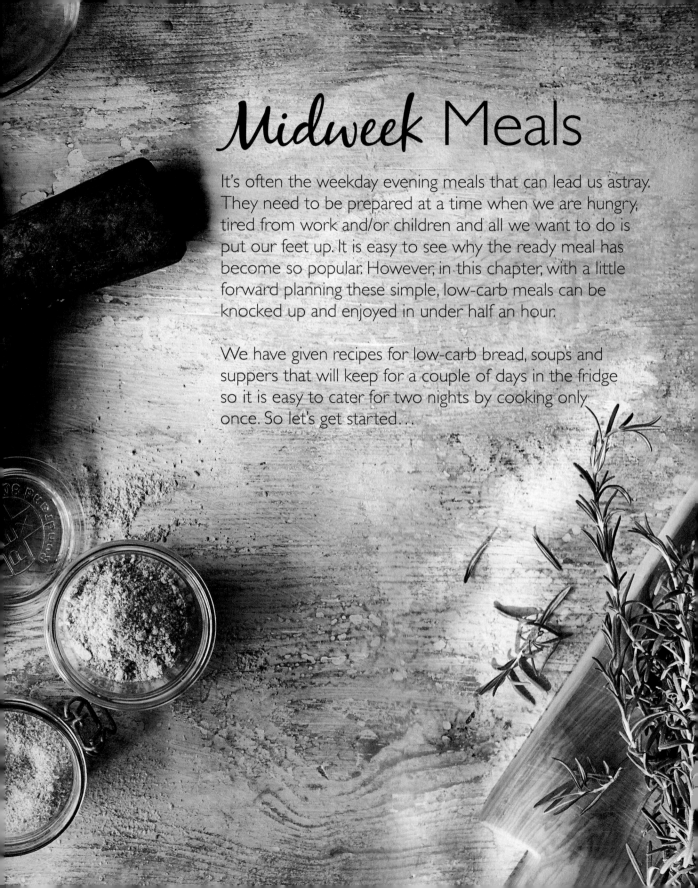

Midweek Meals

It's often the weekday evening meals that can lead us astray. They need to be prepared at a time when we are hungry, tired from work and/or children and all we want to do is put our feet up. It is easy to see why the ready meal has become so popular. However, in this chapter, with a little forward planning these simple, low-carb meals can be knocked up and enjoyed in under half an hour.

We have given recipes for low-carb bread, soups and suppers that will keep for a couple of days in the fridge so it is easy to cater for two nights by cooking only once. So let's get started…

Spinach & Pea Soup

SERVES 6

900g–1kg (2lb–2lb 4oz) frozen spinach

150g (5½oz) frozen peas

50g (1¾oz) butter

1 medium onion, roughly chopped

2 fat garlic cloves, roughly chopped

1 teaspoon grated nutmeg

1 litre (1¾ pints) hot chicken or vegetable stock

6 tablespoons double cream

salt and freshly ground black pepper

To serve (optional)

crumbled feta cheese

goat's cheese

poached eggs

crispy bacon or shredded cooked ham

Per serving (with no additions) 12.4g net carbs, 6.2g fibre, 12.1g protein, 17g fat, 263kcal

This bright green soup is very easy to make and delicious as it is or with one or two of the additions below. Peas give natural sweetness and body to the soup; I have used them in place of a potato, which would usually be used to thicken but is higher in carbs. I always have frozen spinach in my freezer but by all means use fresh spinach instead, you will need about 1.5kg (3lb 5oz). After a good wash, add the fresh spinach to the soup along with the peas. For a bigger meal, enjoy the soup with a couple of poached eggs or a low-carb Bap (page 110).

Put the frozen spinach and peas in a microwavable bowl and microwave on full power for 10 minutes or until defrosted and warm. It doesn't matter if there are a few icy bits left.

Fry the onion and garlic in the butter in a large saucepan over a medium heat. Add 1 teaspoon of salt and the nutmeg to the pan with plenty of freshly ground black pepper.

Drain most of the water from the spinach and peas in a colander, breaking the cubes up with a wooden spoon. Add the spinach and peas to the pan and stir through. Pour in the stock and bring to the boil.

Use a stick blender or a liquidizer to blend the soup until smooth. Return to the pan, then stir in 4 tablespoons of the cream over a medium-high heat. Taste the soup and add seasoning or nutmeg to taste. Pour into warm bowls and swirl through the remaining cream. Add a twist of black pepper and any of the additions you like, then serve.

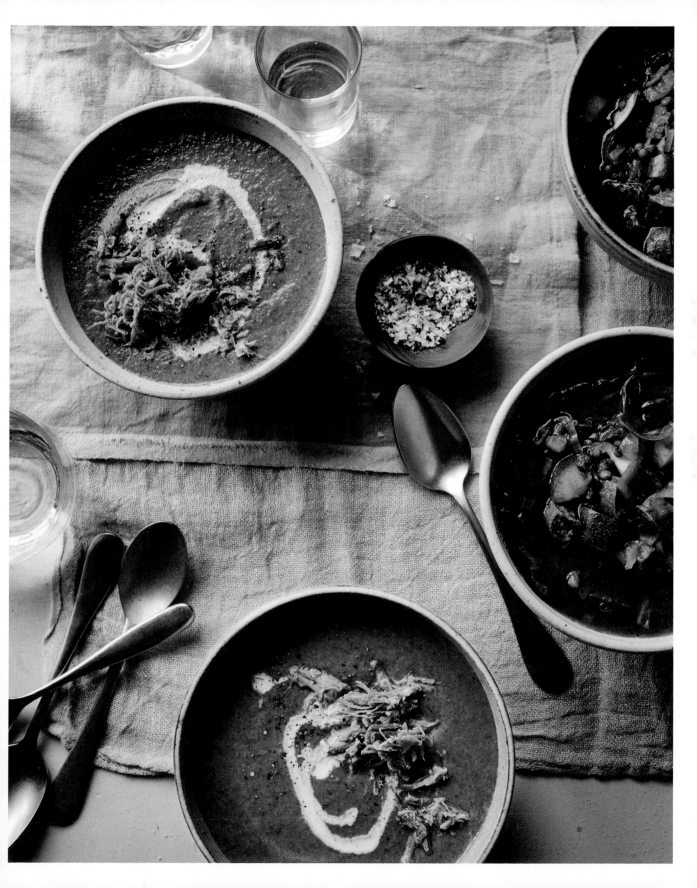

Chilean Chorizo Soup

SERVES 4

2 tablespoons extra virgin olive oil

200g (7oz) leeks or onions, roughly chopped

100g (3½oz) chorizo

1 red pepper

1 medium courgette, roughly chopped

240g (8½oz) cooked green lentils, black or borlotti beans or chickpeas (drained weight)

1 teaspoon dried oregano

½ teaspoon chilli flakes

½ teaspoon ground cumin

400g (14oz) can chopped tomatoes

1 bag baby spinach (optional)

salt and freshly ground black pepper

Per serving 16.3g net carbs, 6.3g fibre, 12.3g protein, 13.8g fat, 256kcal

My Chilean friend Cristina told me about this quick-to-prepare, healthy soup made from chorizo, lentils and vegetables (see the photo on previous page). It is a versatile staple that she makes weekly with whatever vegetables are in season. It also works as a vegetable-based stew or side dish if you add less water. I love the fact that the chorizo gives instant flavour and warmth to the soup. To bump up the protein, enjoy it with the low-carb Focaccia Sticks (page 110) or a couple of soft-boiled eggs.

Fry the leeks in the oil in a wide-based frying pan or saucepan while you prepare the chorizo. I find the easiest way to do this is to make a cut along the length of chorizo and peel the skin off. Cut it in half lengthwise, and again, then hold these four long strips together and cut into 1cm (½in) cubes. Add the chorizo to the pan.

Next, cut the pepper into 1cm (½in) dice and add to the pan followed by the courgette. Stir through and continue to cook for 5 minutes before adding the lentils and spices. Add the tomatoes, then fill the can with warm water and add this too. Bring to the boil, then reduce the heat to medium and cook for 10 minutes; if you prefer a thinner soup, add more water as necessary. Season to taste with salt and plenty of pepper. Stir in the spinach, if using, and serve straight away.

Creamy Vegetable Soup

SERVES 4

1.5 litres (2¾ pints) chicken, meat or vegetable stock

700g (1lb 9oz) assorted vegetables, such as broccoli, cauliflower, celery, courgettes, onions, spring onions, turnip, celeriac and swede

4 tablespoons double cream or Greek yogurt (optional)

salt and freshly ground black pepper

To serve (optional)

1 tablespoon chopped chives

a drizzle of extra virgin olive oil

100g (3½oz) crumbled feta or goat's cheese, or grated Parmesan cheese

8 rashers of cooked smoked bacon, chopped

Per serving 17.1g net carbs, 5g fibre, 13.5g protein, 12g fat, 245kcal

I always thought you had to fry a base of vegetables to make soup until I was shown this method in Bulgaria by Svetlana Nikolova. I was really surprised by the delicious flavour of something so simple. Now I love to make this recipe with the odds and ends from my fridge. I use up broccoli and cauliflower stalks, bendy carrots and celery, celery leaves, courgettes, onions, spring onions, turnip, celeriac and whatever else comes to hand. Celeriac and swede add body to the soup as well as an earthy, spicy flavour which I love. Serve it simply as it is or adorn it with one of the additions below.

Pour the stock into a large saucepan and bring to the boil. Chop the vegetables roughly but with a little thought. Start with the harder root vegetables, such as carrots and swede, peeling and chopping them into thin discs or cubes no bigger than 5mm (¼in). Add them to the pan as soon as they are chopped.

Onions can be cut into 8 wedges and thrown into the pot next as they cook quickly. Then move on to the watery vegetables such as celery and courgettes – these can be cut last and a little larger to save time. Add them to the pan.

Cook the soup for about 15 minutes or until the vegetables are soft. Eat the soup as it is or blend with a stick blender or liquidizer until smooth. Return to the pan to warm over a high heat, then add the cream, if using, and season to taste. Serve straight away as it is or with one of the suggested toppings.

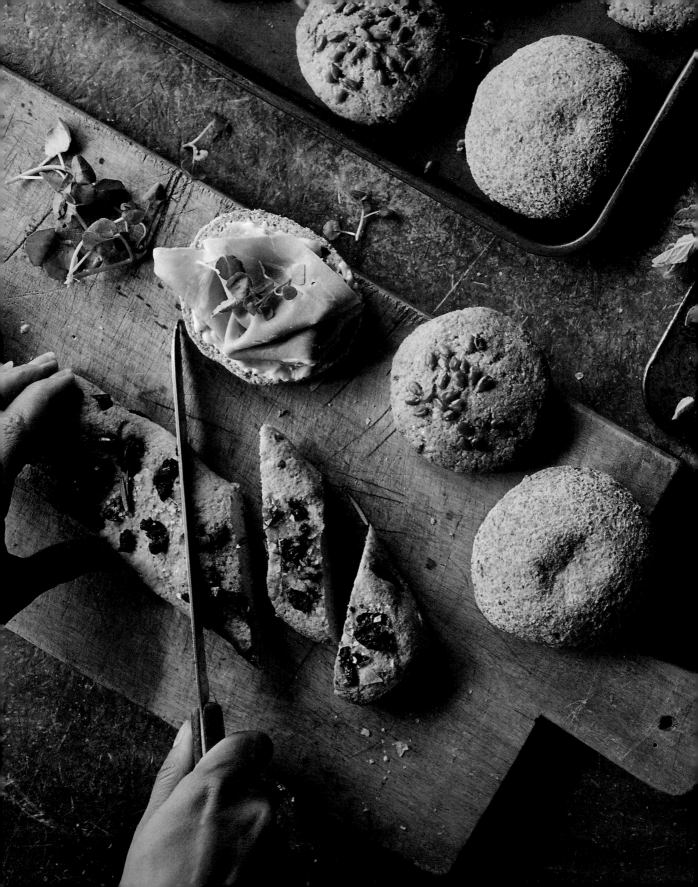

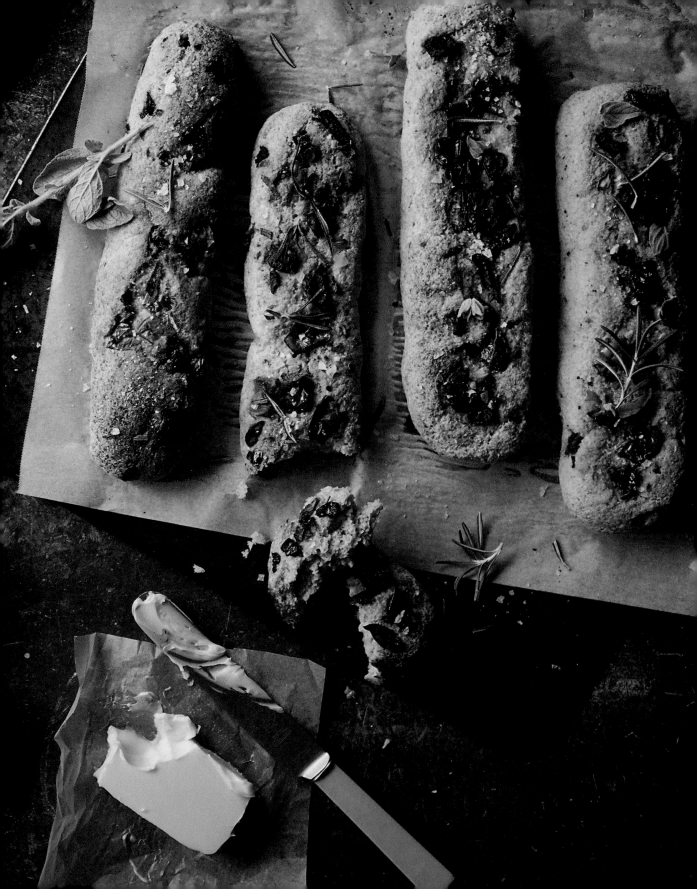

Quick Brown Bread

**MAKES 6 BAPS OR
4 FLAT FOCACCIA STICKS**

olive oil, for greasing

130g (4½oz) ground almonds

30g (1oz) coconut flour

20g (¾oz) coarse psyllium husk

60g (2¼oz) ground golden flaxseed

2 teaspoons baking powder

1 heaped teaspoon salt

3 eggs

1 tablespoon seeds (optional)

sprigs of rosemary (optional)

sea salt flakes (optional)

**Per plain bap or half a focaccia
stick** 13g total carbs, 9.3g fibre, 9.6g
protein, 19g fat, 260kcal

This brown bread is similar to soda bread. It has plenty of flavour, fibre and cooks quickly if you keep the various shapes shallow in depth. The dough can be made into slightly flattened bread rolls, which we call baps, or focaccia sticks and flavoured with nuts, seeds, herbs, chopped sun-dried tomatoes, olives and cheese or used for the Pizza Pronto on page 168. (See the baking hacks on lowcarbtogether.com for more on ingredients, what they do, where to source them and troubleshooting.)

Do try to find golden flaxseed (and grind it yourself on a high-speed blender) and blonde psyllium husk for a good colour but the flavour will be the same with dark brown flaxseed and brown psyllium. This recipe uses coarse psyllium husk, which is cheaper and comes in larger quantities than the powder packaged for medicinal use. If you only have the fine powder, then use the same weight.

Preheat the oven to 220°C/200°C fan/425°F/gas mark 7 and grease a baking tray with a little oil.

Mix the dry ingredients together in a large bowl. Add the eggs and 250ml (9fl oz) water and stir through with a large spoon. When the dough is well combined, use your hands to bring it into a ball. It will thicken all the time as the water is absorbed. Divide the dough according to the instructions opposite and shape using lightly oiled hands.

To make the baps

Roll the dough into 6 balls between your palms, then flatten them into baps about 8cm (3¼in) across and no more than 2cm (¾in) in height. Transfer them to the prepared baking tray, placed at least 4cm (1½in) apart. Press a few seeds into each one, if using.

To make the focaccia sticks

Grease a work surface with a little oil. Divide the dough into 4 and roll out each piece into sausage about 24cm (9½in) long and 3cm (1¼in) thick. Lay the focaccia sticks on the baking tray at least 4cm (1½in) apart and flatten them to about 2cm (¾in) thick. Press a few rosemary needles into each stick and scatter with salt flakes, if using.

Cook the baps and focaccia sticks for 18–22 minutes or until golden brown and firm to the touch.

Additions

Add one or a mixture of these to the dough before shaping:

● *Cheese – 60g (2¼oz) grated Parmesan or other hard cheese*

● *Walnut – 100g (3½oz) chopped walnuts*

● *Herbs – 6 teaspoons of finely chopped fresh or 4 teaspoons of dried herbs such as oregano, thyme, rosemary.*

● *Sun-dried tomato and olive – 60g (2¼oz) chopped sun-dried tomatoes and 40g (1½oz) stoned, roughly chopped olives*

Steak & Chips with Garlic & Rosemary Butter

SERVES 2

1 small swede, weighing about 600g/1lb 5oz, peeled and cut into 1cm (½in) chips

25g (1oz) butter

2 garlic cloves, lightly crushed

2 sprigs rosemary

2 ribeye or sirloin steaks, weighing about 230g (8oz) each and 1.5cm (⅝in) thick

salt and freshly ground black pepper

Per serving 15.5g net carbs, 9g fibre, 28g protein, 9g fat, 207kcal

This is our son Flavio's way of cooking steak; he doesn't like anything to distract from the flavour of the meat other than a hint of garlic and rosemary. We serve this with steamed vegetables (page 128) or a green salad (page 57) and I like a spoonful of mustard alongside. By using swede instead of potato, you can still enjoy steak and chips on a low-carb diet.

Boil the swede in salted water for about 20 minutes or until tender. Drain and set aside.

Heat a large frying pan over a high heat and add the butter, garlic and rosemary sprigs. When hot, add the steaks and season the top sides with salt and plenty of black pepper. Fry for about 2 minutes on each side for rare and 3 minutes on each side for medium. Turn the steaks and season the other side. Tilt the pan and spoon the butter over the steaks as you cook them.

Remove the steaks from the pan and set aside to rest on a board or warm plate, tipping half of the butter over the top. Keep the pan over a medium-high heat and add the swede. Season and fry the chips for 3–4 minutes or until lightly browned all over. Serve straight away with the steaks.

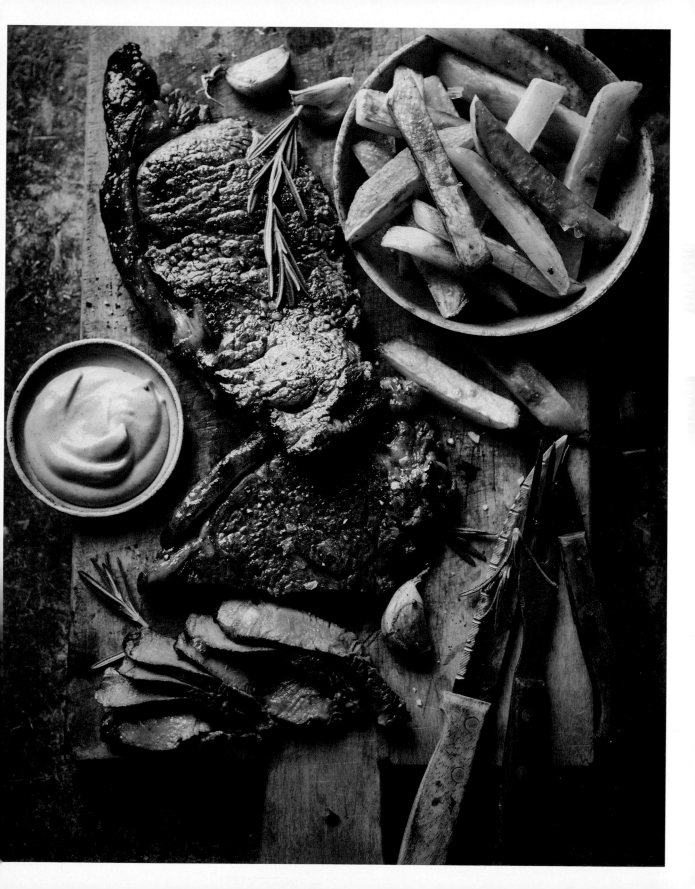

Lamb Steaks, Lentils & Turkish Salad

SERVES 4

12 tablespoons dripping or olive oil, for frying

1 onion, finely sliced

400g (14oz) can cooked green lentils, drained and rinsed

4 lamb steaks, weighing about 600g (1lb 5oz)

salt and freshly ground black pepper

For the Turkish salad

juice of ½ lemon, to taste

2 tablespoons pomegranate molasses

2 tablespoons extra virgin olive oil

1 teaspoon sumac (optional)

4 round tomatoes or a handful of cherry tomatoes

3 small cucumbers or ½ long cucumber

4 spring onions or 1 small onion

a small handful of crunchy salad leaves, such as Romaine, Iceberg or Little Gem lettuce or purslane or watercress

a large handful of one or a mixture of dill, mint leaves, coriander or flat-leaf parsley, chopped

a little finely chopped, spicy green chilli or chilli flakes, to taste (optional)

Per serving of lamb and lentils
10.5g net carbs, 3.8g fibre, 28g protein, 16.1g fat, 311kcal
Per serving of salad 10g net carbs, 2.4g fibre, 1.9g protein, 7.1g fat, 115kcal

For our last summer holiday, we stayed in a hotel on the coast of Turkey. Every day I watched the chefs prepare salad, flashing smiles and blades as I pointed to what I wanted included. They rolled up leaves and huge handfuls of herbs and sliced down without looking. They added garlic, sumac and chilli if you wanted but essential to the flavours were sweet pomegranate molasses and sharp lemon. Don't worry if you don't have one of the ingredients for the salad as there are plenty of others to make up for it. The leaves should add crunch, so use lettuces such as Romaine, iceberg or Little Gem, or purslane or watercress. The salad is great with everything, so once you've mastered it, then try it with fish, meat, chicken or eggs.

Heat the dripping in a frying pan over a medium heat and fry the onion with some seasoning for about 10 minutes until lightly browned and softened.

Meanwhile, make the salad by mixing together the lemon juice, pomegranate molasses, oil and sumac, if using, in a serving bowl and season to taste. Now get chopping, but don't spend ages doing this, a rough cut is fine. Use a serrated knife to cut the tomatoes into dice. Peel the cucumber and dice it; there is no need to deseed it. Line up a row of spring onions and chop them together into fine dice. Add the chopped ingredients to the dressing as you go.

I find the easiest way to cut the lettuce is to lay down the leaves and put the herbs on top (including the stalks, apart from the tough mint stems). Roll them up and hold down with one hand as you chop with the other, cutting them into fine shreds. Toss the salad together, add the chilli, and taste once more for seasoning.

When the onions are soft, add the lentils and stir through to heat for a couple of minutes. Tip the onions and lentils on to warm serving plates and set aside somewhere warm. Keep the pan to cook the lamb.

Season the lamb steaks all over and fry them over a medium-high heat for 2 minutes on each side for medium, or a little longer if you prefer them well done. Put the lamb on top of the lentils and serve with the salad alongside.

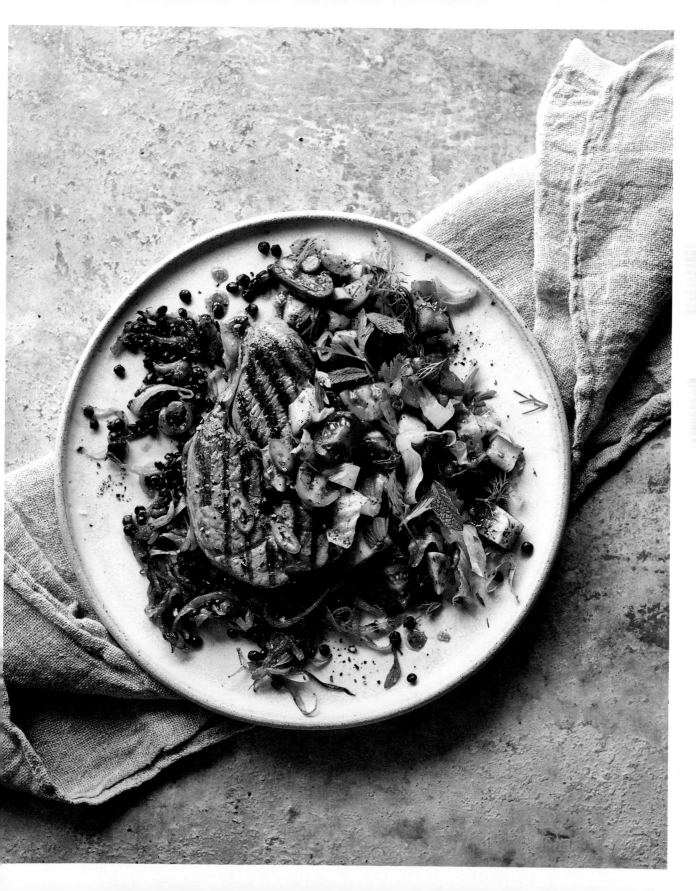

Fajitas & Creamy Guacamole

SERVES 4

1 teaspoon hot chilli powder

1 teaspoon smoked sweet paprika

1 teaspoon ground cumin

500g (1lb 2oz) beef steaks, such
    as sirloin, rump or skirt

1 red pepper

1 medium onion

3 tablespoons extra virgin olive oil

1 garlic clove, grated

salt

For the creamy guacamole

1 avocado

2 heaped tablespoons Greek yogurt

juice of 1 lime

a small handful of coriander leaves,
    finely chopped

½ teaspoon chilli flakes or chopped red
    or green chilli, to taste

To serve

Romaine or Little Gem lettuce leaves

50g (1¾oz) grated mature Cheddar
    cheese or crumbled feta cheese

Per serving 6.3g net carbs, 5.5g fibre,
42.8g protein, 28g fat, 457kcal

Versatile fajitas can be made with any meat. You can use top-quality sirloin steak, less expensive rump or economical skirt steak, or substitute red meat for sliced chicken or turkey. For a veggie version, use strips of aubergine instead. Enjoy as they are or with a dressed salad or large lettuce leaves instead of tortilla wraps. I like to serve this on a large wooden chopping board so everyone can help themselves.

Mix the spices together with 1 teaspoon of salt in a small bowl and then rub the mixture all over the meat. Set aside on a plate.

Warm a serving dish for the vegetables and steak in a low oven or microwave.

Slice the pepper and onion into thin half-moons. Heat half the oil in a large frying pan and fry the vegetables over a medium-high heat for about 8 minutes or until softened and lightly browned.

Meanwhile, make the guacamole by spooning out the flesh from the avocado and using a fork to mash it with the remaining ingredients. (You can also do this in a small food processor if you prefer.) Add salt to taste. Transfer to a small bowl and set aside.

Tip the peppers and onions into the warm serving dish.

Add the remaining oil to the pan over a high heat and when hot add the steaks. Fry for 2 minutes a side for rare and 3 minutes on each side for medium. Transfer them to a clean chopping board to rest for a few minutes.

Lay the lettuce leaves on a large serving plate or chopping board. Add the guacamole bowl and a pile of grated cheese. Slice the steaks into 5mm- (¼in-)thick strips and add to the peppers and onions, along with any cooking juices. Add this bowl to the serving board and serve straight away.

Pork & Mustard with Celeriac Mash

SERVES 4

1 tablespoon extra virgin olive oil

25g (1oz) butter

4 x 2cm- (¾in)-thick pork steaks, weighing about 400g (14oz)

1 onion, finely sliced into half-moons

100ml (3½fl oz) dry white wine

2 teaspoons white wine vinegar or any other vinegar

100ml (3½fl oz) hot vegetable, chicken or meat stock

100ml (3½fl oz) double cream

2 tablespoons Dijon mustard

a small handful of flat-leaf or curly parsley, roughly chopped (optional)

salt and freshly ground black pepper

For the celeriac mash

600g (1lb 5oz) celeriac, peeled and diced into 2cm (¾in) pieces

50g (1¾oz) butter, plus extra to serve

75–100ml (2½–3½fl oz) whole milk

½ teaspoon salt

½ teaspoon ground nutmeg (optional)

30g (1oz) Parmesan cheese, finely grated

Per serving of pork 3.1g net carbs, 0.6g fibre, 24.2g protein, 41.1g fat, 493kcal
Per serving of mash 13g net carbs, 2.7g fibre, 5g protein, 13.2g fat, 195kcal

Pork steaks are inexpensive and quick to cook, and we love this piquant creamy sauce over them. The secret is to cook the steaks quickly and let them rest. We love them on celeriac mash, but they are also good with spinach or green beans. Celeriac mash contains 4g carbs per serving compared to potato mash which has 24g. Celeriac is good with meat as well as fish, fried eggs and sausages. You can use a potato masher but a food processor or stick blender gives the creamy mash that we all love. Any leftovers keep well in the fridge and make a good base for eggs the next day. Other vegetables such as pumpkin, swede, Brussels sprouts, broccoli or cauliflower also make a good mash.

Steam or boil the celeriac in plenty of boiling salted water for 15 minutes or until tender. Drain the celeriac through a sieve or colander and set this over the saucepan for later.

Meanwhile, melt the oil and butter in the large frying pan over a medium-high heat. Put the pork steaks into the pan and season the tops with salt and pepper. Cook for 3 minutes, then turn and season while they cook for a further 3 minutes. Transfer the chops to a plate and set aside.

Return the pan to the heat and add the onion with a little seasoning and fry in the remaining fat for 5–7 minutes over a medium-high heat, stirring occasionally, until softened.

While the onion is cooking, blend the celeriac with the remaining ingredients for the mash in a food processor or with a stick blender until you have a soft, smooth mash. Taste and adjust the seasoning as necessary. Spoon back into the saucepan and put over a low heat to warm through. Stir often to prevent it catching.

Pour the wine and vinegar into the pan with the onion, increase the heat and let it bubble and reduce for 2 minutes. Stir in the stock and bring to the boil, scraping any brown bits off the bottom of the pan. Add the cream and mustard and stir through for a couple of minutes, allowing the sauce to bubble and thicken. Return the chops to the pan to reheat for 3 minutes, spooning the sauce over them. Season to taste.

Serve the pork on warm plates with the sauce over them and the mash on the side. Scatter over the parsley, if using.

Midweek Meaty Pilaff

SERVES 4

3 tablespoons extra virgin olive oil

1 onion or leek, finely chopped

1 fat garlic clove, crushed

200g (7oz) lamb mince

approx. 240g (8½oz) chicken livers or merguez sausages

400g (14oz) cauliflower, riced

1–2 tablespoons harissa paste

1 teaspoon ground cumin

100ml (3½fl oz) meat stock, hot water or leftover gravy

2 tablespoons finely chopped herbs, such as coriander, dill or flat-leaf parsley

salt and freshly ground black pepper

Per serving 7g net carbs, 2.5g fibre, 30.1g protein, 21.8g fat, 351kcal

Think of this as a meaty, one-pan midweek meal that uses mince, liver or sausages and cauliflower rice as a base. Swap out any of the uncooked meat for leftover cooked meat and use up any gravy instead of the stock. Use lamb, beef or pork mince and any liver. Look for high-meat-content sausages that don't contain starch, such as merguez, Toulouse or Italian varieties. The pilaff is great finished with a lot of herbs; I use a mixture from the fridge and what is in the garden, but you could scatter over a couple of teaspoons of dried thyme or oregano if that is all you have to hand. Do taste your harissa before adding; they differ, some are spicy or salty and others are mild.

Pour the oil into a large frying pan over a medium heat, add the onion and sweat it for 5 minutes. Add a little seasoning, the garlic and mince and stir through to break up the mince.

Cut any tough, white, connective tissue away from the chicken livers and roughly chop them or, if using sausages, chop them into bite-sized pieces. Increase the heat and add the livers or sausages and cook for 7–10 minutes until brown all over and cooked through.

Stir in the cauliflower rice, harissa and cumin and stock, cover and cook for 5 minutes over a medium heat. Check a couple of times, you may need more stock or a splash of water if things look dry. You should see the cauliflower rice change from bright white grains to soft creamy-coloured ones. Taste and add seasoning if necessary. Fold in the herbs and serve straight from the pan into warm bowls.

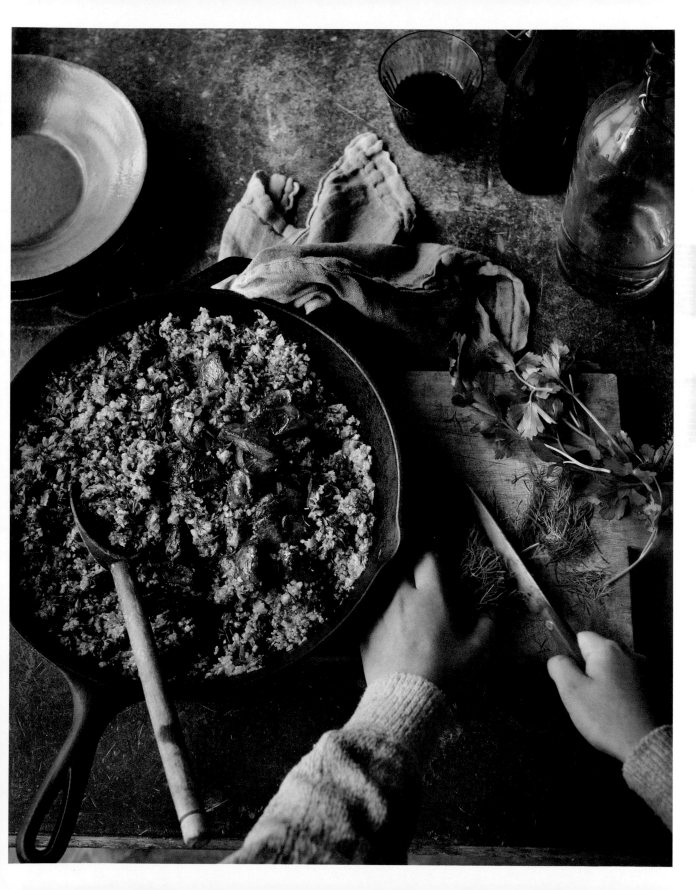

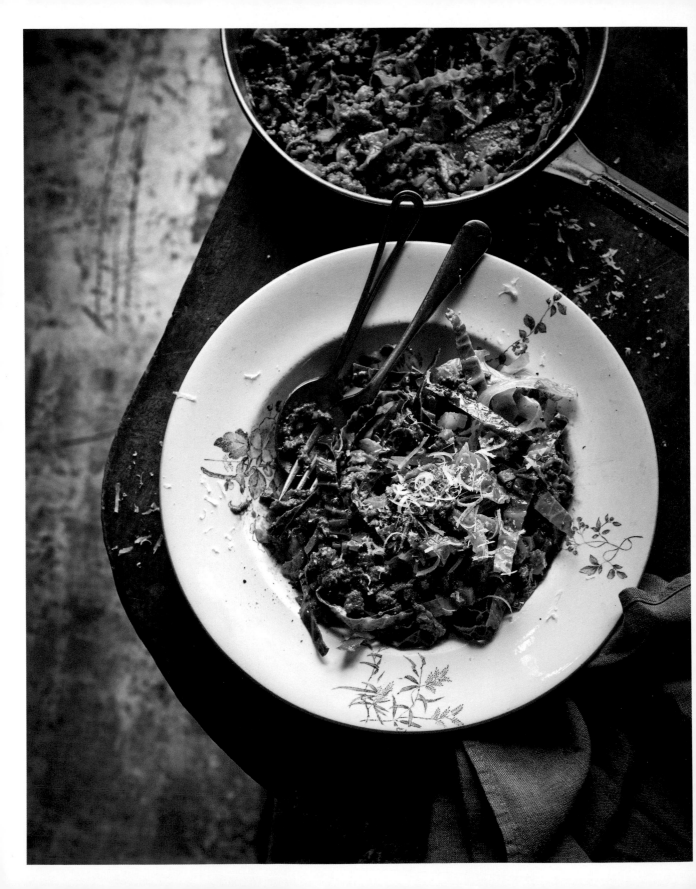

Quick Ragù on Savoy Pezzi

SERVES 6

4 tablespoons extra virgin olive oil

2 garlic cloves, lightly crushed

1 onion, finely chopped

1 medium carrot, scrubbed
    finely chopped

2 celery sticks, finely chopped

1 sprig of rosemary or thyme or
    1 bay leaf

500g (1lb 2oz) 15% fat beef mince

100ml (3½fl oz) red wine

400g (14oz) can chopped Italian, plum
    or cherry tomatoes

1 tablespoon tomato purée

3 tablespoons double cream (optional)

15g (½oz) Parmesan cheese,
    finely grated

salt and freshly ground black pepper

For the Savoy pezzi (serves 2)

300g (10½oz) Savoy, sweetheart or
    other cabbage

20g (¾oz) butter

Per serving of ragù 4.2g net carbs,
2.1g fibre, 17.6g protein, 25g fat,
315kcal

Per serving of pezzi 0.4g net carbs,
3.3g fibre, 7.6g protein, 17g fat,
208kcal

In *The Reverse Your Diabetes Cookbook* we referred to a perfect swap for pasta as "pezzi", which translates as "pieces" in Italian. The term refers to roughly torn pieces of any cabbage that are cooked quickly with butter, salt and pepper until they wilt and form a delicious low-carb base for pasta sauces. This makes enough pezzi for two; it is perfect with the ragù and many other traditional pasta sauces and also makes a simple side dish for sausages, roast meat or eggs. Simply double or triple the recipe for four and six portions.

Normally the Italian ragù that we serve in our restaurants takes up to 5 hours to make but here we've created a 30-minute version that would make any Italian mamma proud. The ragù is perfect to make in a large batch like this as it will keep in the fridge for up to 5 days and freezes for up to 3 months.

Heat the oil in a large frying pan over a medium-high heat and fry the garlic, onion, carrot, celery and herbs for 7 minutes or until softened.

Increase the heat, add the mince to the pan and fry until browned, breaking it up with a wooden spoon. Any water in the mince should come out at this point, so when the mince is starting to look dry, add the wine and bring to the boil. Let it reduce for 2 minutes. Then add the tomatoes and tomato purée and bring the ragù to the boil. Cook for a further 15 minutes and then stir in the cream, if using.

Meanwhile, make the Savoy pezzi. Remove any thick, tough stems, damaged leaves and the hard core from the cabbage. Tear or cut the leaves into pieces about 5–7cm (2–3in) across or roll up the leaves and cut them into ribbons similar to tagliatelle. Put into a microwavable bowl with the butter, 4 tablespoons of water, salt and pepper. Microwave on full power for 5–7 minutes, covered with a plate, stirring once halfway through cooking.

Alternatively, put the cabbage ribbons in a medium saucepan with the butter, 4 tablespoons of water and seasoning and cover with a lid. Cook over a medium heat for 5–15 minutes or until it is almost transparent and tender; this will depend upon your type of cabbage. Kale only takes about 5 minutes. Drain and keep warm until the sauce is ready.

To serve, heat enough ragù for two in a saucepan and stir in the drained cabbage. Top with the Parmesan and a twist of black pepper.

Stuffed Mushrooms

SERVES 4

8 portobello mushrooms, weighing
*   about 500g (1lb 2oz)*

a knob of butter, for greasing

1 medium leek or onion

400g (14oz) minced beef, lamb or
*   pork or sausage meat*

50g (1¾oz) Parmesan cheese, grated

2 teaspoons Worcestershire sauce

salt and freshly ground black pepper

Per serving with beef mince
10.9g net carbs, 1.8g fibre, 25.6g
protein, 23g fat, 350kcal

I always find huge mushrooms impressive and can't help thinking of ways of using them as containers for a myriad of stuffings. Use any minced meat you like or split open a few high-meat-content sausages and use the sausage meat. For a vegetarian version, use drained cooked beans, such as cannellini or borlotti beans, instead. Do experiment with flavourings such as thyme, garlic or parsley, or try topping them with grated Cheddar or blue cheese instead of the Parmesan. Serve with green vegetables or a salad or try them with the herb & cheese cauliflower couscous (page 124).

Preheat the oven to 220°C/200°C fan/425°F/gas mark 7.

Remove the stalks from the mushrooms and put them into a food processor. Put the mushroom tops in a greased ovenproof dish. Roughly chop the leek and add this to the food processor, then whizz until finely chopped. (Alternatively, you can do all the chopping by hand.)

Transfer the mushroom and leek mixture to a bowl and mix together with the mince, cheese, Worcestershire sauce and some seasoning (omit this if you are using seasoned sausage meat). Divide the mixture evenly between the cavities of the mushrooms, flattening the tops down a little so they all have the same depth and cooking time. Any leftover mixture can be rolled into balls and cooked alongside the mushrooms.

Cook for 10–15 minutes or until the meat is cooked through and the mushrooms are tender. Serve with any juices from the dish and a side dish such as watercress, cauliflower couscous (page 124) or celeriac mash (page 117).

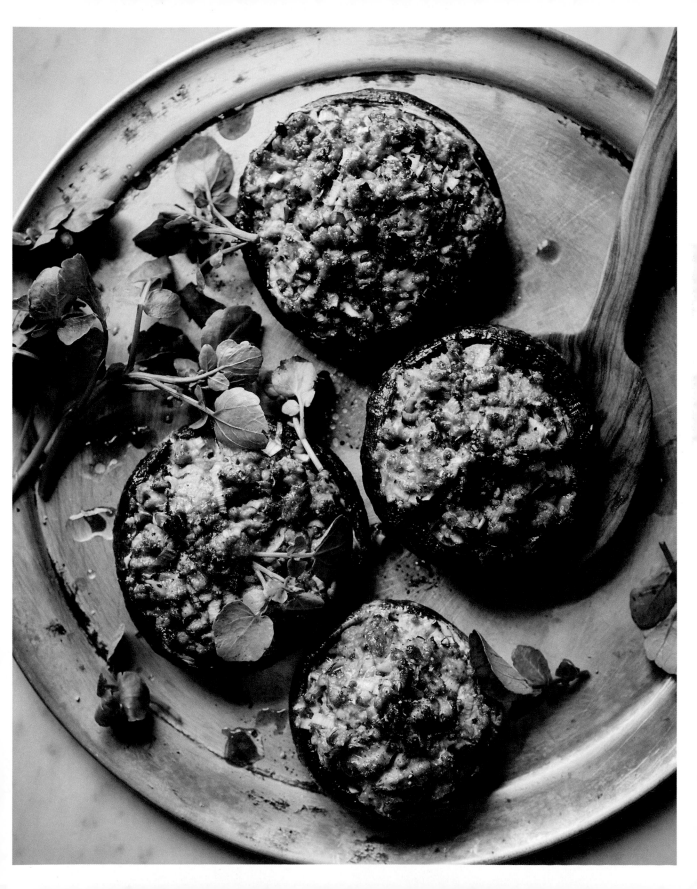

Cauliflower Rice

SERVES 4

400g (14oz) cauliflower (flower,
*   stalk and leaves), broccoli or sprouts*

2 tablespoons extra virgin olive oil,
*   ghee, coconut oil, chicken fat or*
*   beef dripping*

1 small onion or leek, or 5 spring onions,
*   finely chopped*

salt and freshly ground black pepper

Per serving 4.4g net carbs, 2.2g fibre,
2.1g protein, 7g fat, 91kcal

To avoid blood sugar spikes from eating rice or couscous, switch to cauliflower rice instead. Once cooked, it keeps in the fridge for 3 days (or in the freezer for up to 3 months).

Cut the head of the cauliflower into large florets and roughly chop the stalk and leaves. Put a third of the cauliflower into a food processor and pulse until finely chopped (it will resemble large grains of rice), making sure you don't end up with a purée. Tip into a bowl and repeat with the remaining two thirds. If you don't have a food processor, coarsely grate the florets and stalk and finely chop the leaves.

Heat the fat in a wok or large frying pan. Fry the onion over a medium heat for 5–7 minutes or until soft. Add the cauliflower rice, season and stir through. Add 75ml (2½fl oz) water, cover and cook over a low heat for about 7 minutes or until just soft, stirring occasionally.

Cauliflower Couscous

SERVES 4

400g (14oz) cauliflower

3 tablespoons extra virgin olive oil,
*   ghee, coconut oil or dripping*

1 small onion or leek, or 5 spring onions,
*   finely chopped*

1 red pepper, cut into finger-width strips

1 fat garlic clove, finely chopped

½ teaspoon chilli flakes (optional)

1 teaspoon ground cumin

1 teaspoon ground turmeric

a small handful of coriander or flat-leaf
*   parsley, leaves roughly chopped,*
*   stems finely chopped*

salt and freshly ground black pepper

Per serving 6.2g net carbs, 2.6g fibre,
2.4g protein, 10.5g fat, 131kcal

Add peppers and a couple of spices to cauliflower rice to transform it into a flavourful couscous-style dish that is perfect with the Stuffed Mushrooms on page 122, any roast meat or grilled fish. We also like it with a couple of soft-boiled eggs and a dollop of Greek yogurt. It keeps well in the fridge for up to 3 days and is easy to reheat in a microwave or frying pan.

Rice the cauliflower as described above and set aside.

Heat the fat in a wok or large frying pan. Fry the onion and pepper over a medium heat for 5–7 minutes or until soft. Add the garlic, chilli, if using, cumin, turmeric and seasoning. Add the cauliflower rice along with 6 tablespoons of water. Cover and cook over a low heat for about 7 minutes or until just soft, stirring occasionally.

When cooked, stir in the herbs and serve straight away.

Gammon Steak, Parsley & Leek Cream

SERVES 2

2 medium leeks (about 300g/10½oz
  pre-prepared weight)

25g (1oz) butter, plus extra for frying

75ml (2½fl oz) double cream

25g (1oz) Parmesan cheese, grated

10g (¼oz) flat-leaf parsley leaves,
  roughly chopped

2 gammon steaks, weighing about
  400g (14oz)

1 tablespoon extra virgin olive oil

2 tomatoes, halved

salt and freshly ground black pepper

Per serving 7.7g net carbs, 2.6g fibre,
43.4g protein, 49g fat, 652kcal

The combination of sweet leeks, cheese and smoky gammon is an absolute winner. We had great fun testing this recipe and thinking how these easy-peasy-cheesy leeks could go with so many other dishes, such as poached eggs, sausages or any food that works with a creamy sauce.

Wash the leeks and make sure there is no mud in the ends, then cut them into 2cm (¾in) widths.

Melt the butter in a frying pan over a medium heat, add the leeks with some seasoning and a splash of water, cover with a lid and fry for 10 minutes. Add the cream, scatter over the Parmesan and stir through. Taste for seasoning, cook for a further couple of minutes and then set aside.

In a separate frying pan, fry the gammon steaks (one at a time if necessary) in the olive oil and a knob of butter until lightly browned on one side, then flip to the other side and do the same. They will only take 3–4 minutes a side. If there is room in the pan, fry the tomatoes on both sides at the same time or cook afterwards until just soft and lightly browned.

Reheat the leeks in their pan and serve over the gammon on warm plates with the tomatoes on the side and any juices from the pan poured over the top.

Shopski Cheese

SERVES 2

15g (½oz) butter, for greasing and dotting on top

1 small onion, finely chopped

100g (3½oz) feta cheese, sliced into 4 pieces

2 tablespoons flat-leaf parsley, finely chopped, or a pinch of dried herbs (optional)

50g (1¾oz) smoked ham or sausage or cooked bacon, diced (optional)

400g (14oz) tomatoes, chopped, or 400g (14oz) can chopped tomatoes

2 eggs

2 hot chillies, finely chopped or chilli flakes added to taste (optional)

salt and freshly ground black pepper

Per serving 8.8g net carbs, 4.3g fibre, 19g protein, 22.4g fat, 323kcal

Shopski means something done in the way that the *shopi* do it. The *shopi* are the west Bulgarians who cook with a *gyuveche*, a pretty earthenware pot with a hole in the top. I have experimented at home with cereal bowls and foil, Le Creuset dishes and old enamel pots and they all work for this dish. You just need to make sure that you have a small, sealed ovenproof container. The difference will be the cooking time as the heat transfers more quickly through metal than it does through pottery. In fact, if you are using a traditional *gyuveche*, then you must put it into the oven cold and then turn the heat on so that it heats up slowly. This isn't necessary with other ovenproof dishes, which can be safely put into a hot oven.

Use your imagination with this dish and add leftover meat and vegetables, roast peppers from a jar and/or salami, but this is the standard version shown to me by *shopi* Svetlana Nikolova. One of the low-carb Baps (page 110) is lovely alongside to scoop up the sauce, or you can add another egg if you are feeling hungry.

Preheat the oven to 220°C/200°C fan/425°F/gas mark 7.

Butter two small ovenproof dishes (see the introduction) generously and then add half the chopped onion into each of them. Then add one piece of feta into each, followed by the parsley and ham, if using, tomatoes, the remaining feta and an egg cracked on one side. Dot over the remaining butter, add a little seasoning and put the chilli on the opposite side to the egg, if using.

Put on the lid or fashion a piece of foil tightly over each one and cook for about 20 minutes or until the eggs are done to your liking. Serve straight away.

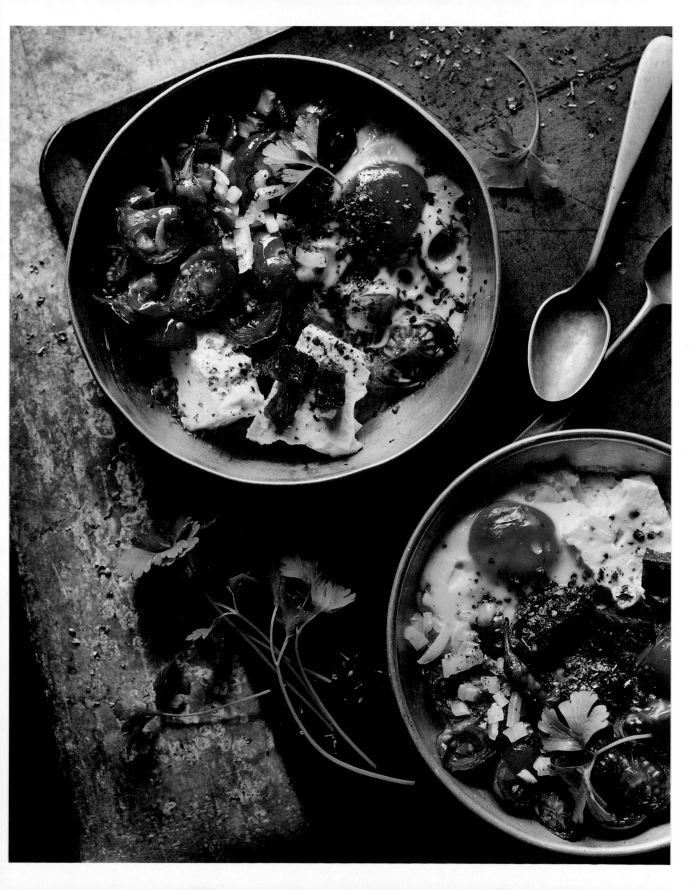

Mustard Chicken with Steamed Vegetables

SERVES 2

1 onion, finely sliced into half-moons

3 tablespoons extra virgin olive oil

4 tablespoons white wine or water

2 sprigs of rosemary

2 tablespoons English mustard

2 medium skinless chicken breasts

salt and freshly ground black pepper

Per serving of chicken and onions
7.5g net carbs, 0.8g fibre, 39.2g protein, 27.5g fat, 463kcal
Per serving of courgettes and carrots 1.8g net carbs, 0.8g fibre, 1.8g protein, 4.4g fat, 61kcal

Flavour suggestions

● 200g (7oz) courgettes and carrots, thinly sliced, with a knob of butter and zest of ½ lemon – 7–10 minutes

● 100g (3½oz) leeks, cut into 1cm (½in) discs, 100g (3½oz) cherry tomatoes together with a knob of butter – 8 minutes

● 300g (10½oz) shredded Savoy cabbage with a knob of ghee and a good pinch of salt, cumin seeds and garam masala – 8–10 minutes

● 300g (10½oz) cauliflower florets with a pinch of black pepper, black onion (nigella) seeds, salt, 1 chopped garlic clove and a knob of butter – 15 minutes

Firstly, yes, I do mean 2 tablespoons of hot, strong, bright yellow English mustard. The heat disappears in the oven, leaving delicious mildly spiced chicken on a bed of sweet roast onions. Steaming vegetables in a parcel intensifies their flavour; children and fussy eaters can prepare their own and just have fun with flavour. We write their names on the parcels.

Preheat the oven to 220°C/200°C fan/425°F/gas mark 7.

Toss the onion with 2 tablespoons of the oil and some seasoning, then divide into 2 piles in an ovenproof dish. Pour over the white wine and lay a rosemary sprig on each pile.

Spoon the mustard into a separate bowl so you aren't going back and forth between the uncooked chicken and the pot. Spread the mustard over both breasts with the back of the spoon. Lay them on top of the onion. Drizzle over the remaining oil and grind over a little pepper.

Cook for 20 minutes or until the chicken is cooked through and pink juices no longer run from the chicken when the thickest part is pierced with a fork. Thicker breasts may take longer to cook. You can also use a probe thermometer to make sure it is at 74°C (165°F) inside.

To make a parcel for the steamed vegetables, cut a piece of baking parchment at least 10cm (4in) larger than the food you are about to cook. Lay the vegetables, seasoning, any oil or butter and herbs or spices in the centre of the parchment. Fold the long ends up to meet each other above the food. Make a fold of both pieces together of about 2cm (¾in) then fold again. Repeat until the fold is about 4cm (1½in) above the food. Now twist each end like a sweet wrapper. Transfer to a baking tray.

The vegetables will take 7–15 minutes depending on their density and size. The more watery, soft vegetables, such as courgettes, take less time than firm carrots, and the finer you cut them, the quicker they will cook. You can press the top of the parcel(s) to feel the give in the vegetables.

Serve your choice of steamed vegetables in the parcel alongside the mustard chicken.

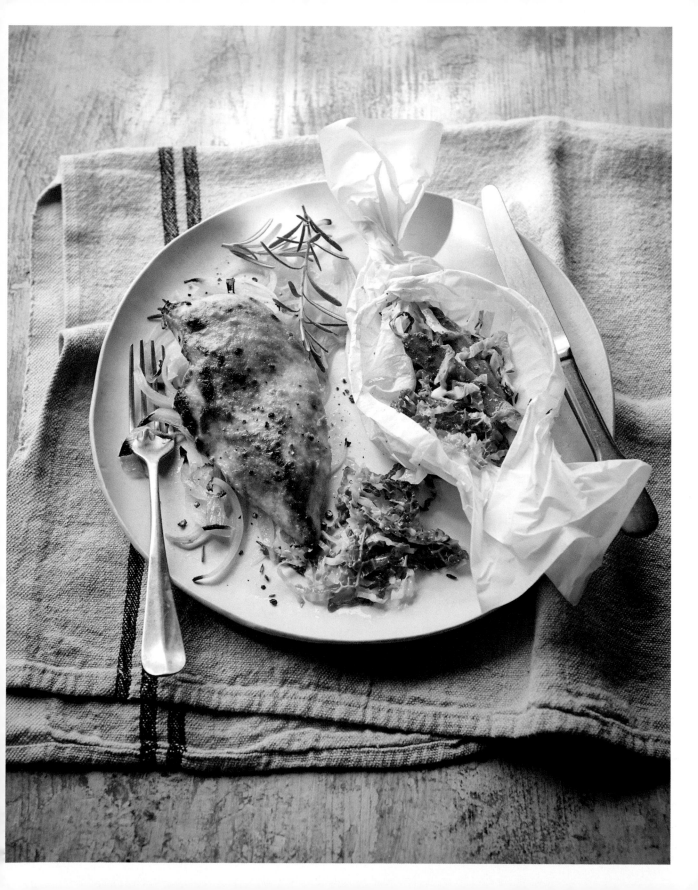

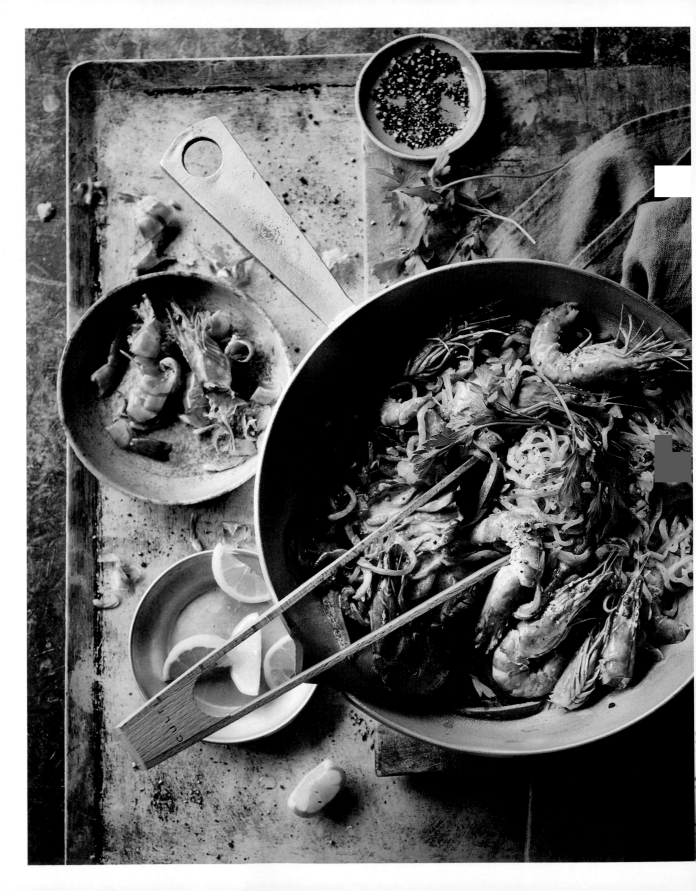

Creamy Paprika Prawns

SERVES 2

170–200g (6–7oz) konjac noodles (drained weight)

2 tablespoons extra virgin olive oil or butter

1 onion, finely sliced into half-moons

½ red pepper, finely sliced

1 garlic clove, finely chopped or crushed

150g (5½oz) frozen or defrosted cooked prawns

1 teaspoon smoked paprika

a pinch of chilli flakes or finely chopped hot chilli

4 tablespoons dry white wine

3 tablespoons double cream

a handful of flat-leaf parsley, roughly chopped (optional)

½ lemon, cut into wedges, to serve

Per serving 4.6g net carbs, 4.3g fibre, 18g protein, 25.7g fat, 354kcal

Frozen cooked or raw prawns are quick and easy options in this dish, where they are flavoured with chilli and garlic. If you can find raw prawns with the heads intact, then these give a proper prawn taste; peel away the shells and tails and leave the heads on. Cook them as in the recipe below, giving them time to turn completely pink. Squeeze the juices from the heads with a wooden spoon as they cook to release more shellfish flavour.

Rinse the noodles under cold water until cool to the touch, drain thoroughly in a sieve over a bowl and set aside.

Heat the oil in a large frying pan over a high heat and when hot add the onion, pepper and garlic. Cook for 5 minutes, stirring frequently, then add the prawns, paprika and chilli. Keep stirring and allow the cooked prawns to heat through or the raw prawns to turn pink. Pour in the wine and cook for a couple of minutes to allow the sauce to reduce. Add the cream and stir through.

Tip the drained noodles into the pan and stir to coat them. Cook for a couple of minutes to heat the noodles and reduce the sauce. Use tongs to divide between two warm bowls and scatter over the parsley, if using. Serve with the lemon wedges.

Peppers & Sardines

SERVES 2

2 red peppers

2 cans of sardines or salmon or tuna, weighing about 175g (6oz)

8 cherry tomatoes, halved

10 black olives, stoned (optional)

8 anchovy fillets in oil (optional)

4 teaspoons baby capers, drained and rinsed (optional)

1 heaped teaspoon dried oregano (optional)

a pinch of chilli flakes (optional)

2 tablespoons extra virgin olive oil

salt and freshly ground black pepper

Per serving 7.5g net carbs, 3.8g fibre, 25.7g protein, 27.3g fat, 390kcal

Pepper halves are brilliant, colourful vessels for a variety of fillings and cook perfectly in 25 minutes. "Optional" appears after many of the ingredients as this is a very adaptable recipe and won't be harmed by the omission of one or two ingredients if you don't have them or don't like them. If you can, buy whole black olives, Taggiasche are perfect, with stones in and remove them by bashing the olive with the flat side of a cook's knife and picking them out. The flavour will be much better than the ready-stoned variety. Look out for baby capers or those in salt as they have less of a vinegary taste than the larger ones.

Preheat the oven to 220°C/200°C fan/425°F/gas mark 7.

Halve the pepper lengthways through the stalk. Pick out the white membrane and seeds. Drain the sardines in a sieve.

Put the peppers in an ovenproof dish or roasting tray. Layer up the sardines, tomatoes and olives, anchovies, capers, oregano and chilli flakes, if using, into each pepper cavity with a little seasoning (as the anchovies are salty) and oil as you go. Finish with a drizzle of oil and cook for 20–25 minutes or until the peppers are tender and the filling is piping hot. Serve alone or with the green salad on page 57.

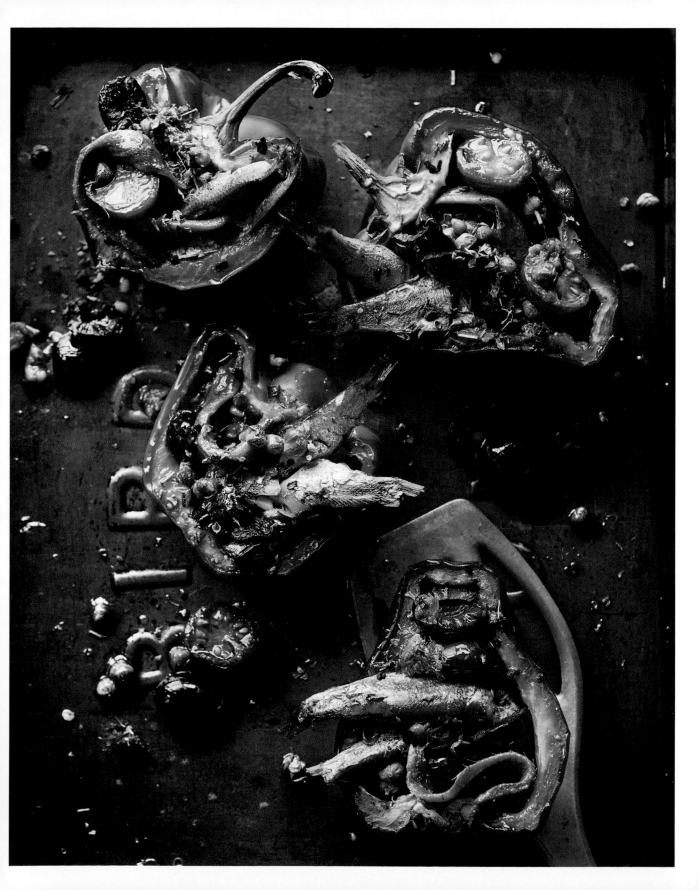

Fish & Chips

SERVES 2

250g (9oz) celeriac, peeled and cut into
    1cm (½in) chips

1 tablespoon extra virgin olive oil

1 low-carb Bap (page 110)

1 egg

280g (10oz) haddock or other
    sustainable firm white fish, skinned

salt and freshly ground black pepper

For the tartare sauce

2 tablespoons mayonnaise

1 tablespoon capers, rinsed, drained
    and roughly chopped

1 gherkin (finger size), roughly chopped

1 teaspoon lemon juice, plus lemon
    wedges, to serve

Per serving of fish & chips 8g net
carbs, 6.1g fibre, 36.7g protein, 20g
fat, 383kcal
Per serving of tartare sauce 2.9g net
carbs, 0.2g fibre, 0.3g protein, 9.8g fat,
101kcal

The average portion of fish and chips can have up to 69g carbs. To make this version, you need to make the Quick Brown Bread on page 110, but the health benefits and flavour more than make up for it and you will have leftover baps for another day. I have allowed time to make tartare sauce as I love the homemade version but do skip this if you don't have the ingredients. We serve this with a green salad (page 57) or buttered baby spinach.

Preheat the oven to 220°C/200°C fan/425°F/gas mark 7.

Put the celeriac chips on a baking tray and use your fingertips to toss evenly with the oil and some salt and pepper. Spread out in a single layer, pushing the chips to one side to allow room for the fish later. Bake for 13 minutes.

Meanwhile, grate the low-carb bap or whizz in a food processor to make breadcrumbs. Pour them on to a plate and spread out. Break the egg into a shallow bowl and beat with a fork.

If the fish isn't already portioned, cut into two pieces and season evenly with a little salt. Dip into the beaten egg, followed by the breadcrumbs. Lay the fish on a plate and set aside until the chips have cooked for 13 minutes.

Remove the chips from the oven, add the fish to the space you have left for it and cook both for 10–12 minutes or until the fish is cooked through and the chips are soft and golden brown. Remove the tray from the oven as soon as the fish feels firm to the touch and the chips are done.

While they are cooking, make the tartare sauce by mixing all the ingredients together and adding the lemon juice to taste. Cut the remaining lemon into wedges to serve.

Serve the fish, chips and tartare sauce on warm plates and enjoy!

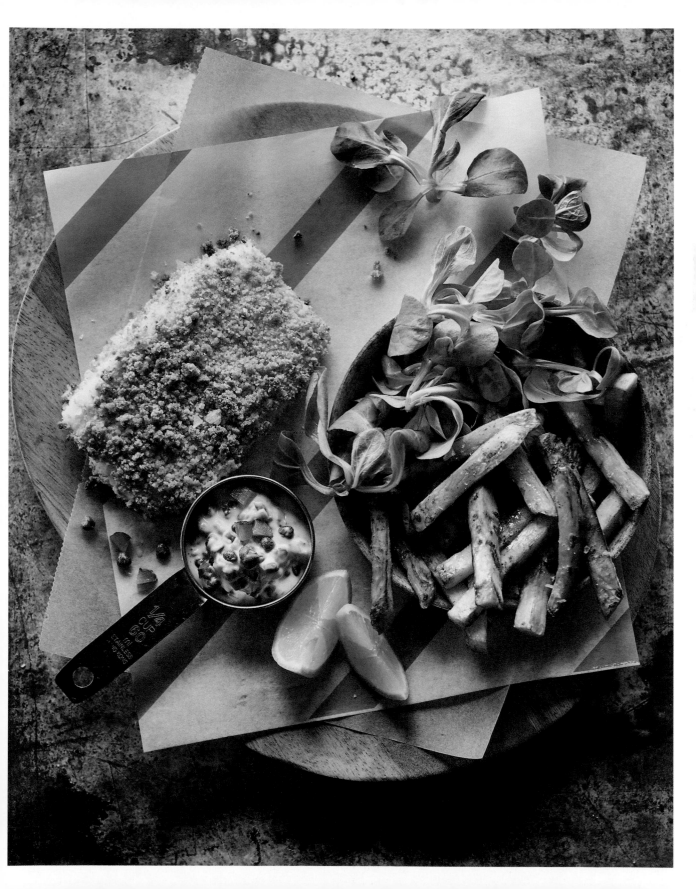

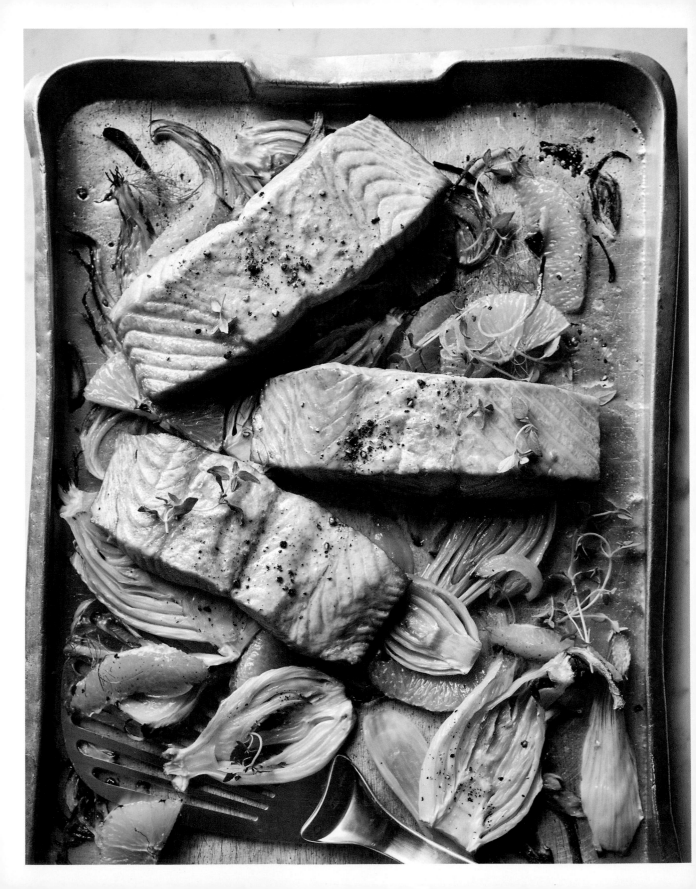

Salmon with Thyme, Orange & Fennel

SERVES 4

approx. 700g (1lb 9oz) fennel bulbs (untrimmed weight)

4 tablespoons extra virgin olive oil

1 medium orange

4 x 120g (4½oz) salmon steaks

1 medium brown onion, sliced into half-moons

4 tablespoons white wine or water (optional)

a few sprigs of thyme or 1 teaspoon dried thyme or rosemary

salt and freshly ground black pepper

Per serving 12.9g net carbs, 6.6g fibre, 33.3g protein, 23.6g fat, 430kcal

If you need cheering up, then this is the dish for you. The bright, clashing colours of the pink salmon, vibrant orange and pale green fennel are as pretty as a picture on the plate and the flavours love each other's company. Rather than waste the tough outer fennel, if there are pale brown areas or tough veins running through the leaves, then remove them with a potato peeler rather than lose the whole piece.

Trim the tough stalks and base away from the fennel, reserving a few feathery green fronds to serve. Cut the bulbs into 1cm (½in) slices from top to base. Cook in boiling water for 5 minutes, then drain in a sieve and set aside.

Preheat the oven to 200°C/180°C fan/400°F/gas mark 6 and brush a roasting tray with a little of the oil.

Use a sharp knife to cut away the peel from the orange, trying to waste as little flesh as possible. Then cut the orange in half and rest each half on a board flat-side down. Cut each half into 6–7 segments.

Season the salmon all over and lay on the prepared tray. Put the drained fennel, onion and orange around the fish and season with salt and pepper. Pour the wine over the vegetables, if using. Drizzle the remaining oil over the fish and scatter the thyme over everything. Bake for 12–15 minutes or until the fish is cooked through.

Serve straight away scattered with the reserved fennel fronds.

Sea Bass with Tarragon

SERVES 2

25g (1oz) butter, plus a knob for frying the fish

4 spring onions, white and green parts, sliced on diagonal, or 1 small onion, finely chopped

100g (3½oz) frozen peas

2 Little Gem lettuce hearts, quartered into wedges

75ml (2½fl oz) dry white wine

50ml (2fl oz) double cream

7g (¼oz) tarragon leaves, stems discarded

1 tablespoon extra virgin olive oil

2 sea bass fillets, skin on

salt and freshly ground black pepper

Per serving 8.1g net carbs, 3.5g fibre, 20.7g protein, 41.12g fat, 519kcal

This recipe is perfect for a date-night in. With the prettiness of the lettuce and peas and the crispy skin of the sea bass it has the look of restaurant food but is easy and quick to make. Light a candle or two, pour a couple of glasses of Chablis and you'll think you've gone out for the evening!

Melt the butter in a large frying pan over a medium–high heat, add the spring onions and some seasoning and fry for about 5 minutes or until soft. Warm 2 serving bowls in a low oven.

Put the peas in a sieve and pour a kettle of just-boiled water over them. Drain and add to the pan with the lettuce wedges. Let the lettuce brown and the peas cook through, then pour in the wine. Let it bubble for a couple of minutes before adding the cream and most of the tarragon (reserving some to serve). Cook for 2 minutes to allow the sauce to reduce. Taste the sauce and adjust the seasoning. You will need a large frying pan to cook the fish, so transfer the vegetables to a bowl if necessary and keep warm. Otherwise leave the pan over a very low heat.

To cook the fish, heat a knob of butter and the oil in a large frying pan over a medium–high heat until it foams. Season the fish fillets all over and add them to the pan skin-side down. Cook for about 5 minutes until the skin crisps and the fish becomes opaque around the edges, then flip them over with a fish slice or spatula and cook on the other side for a minute or two. Check the fillets are cooked through by making sure the flesh is white rather than pinkish raw. Remove the pan from the heat.

Divide the vegetables between the warm bowls and top each one with a sea bass fillet. Scatter over the remaining tarragon, garnish with a twist of black pepper and serve straight away.

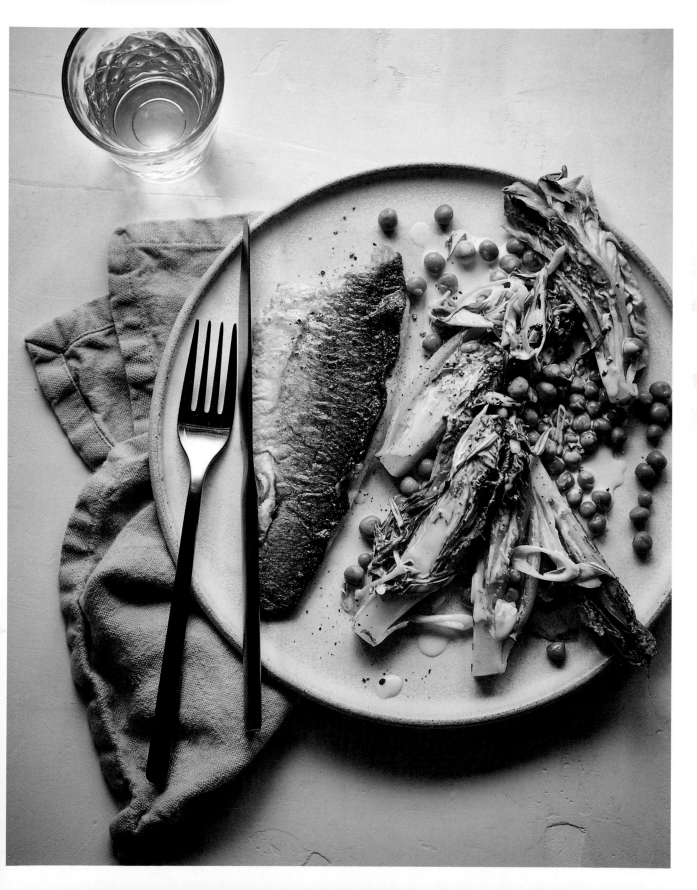

Mackerel & Mustard

SERVES 2

2 tablespoons extra virgin olive oil

1 heaped teaspoon wholegrain or
English mustard

4 tablespoons soured cream, crème
fraîche or Greek yogurt

1 lemon

4 mackerel fillets, weighing about 360g
(12½oz), pin-boned

8 cherry tomatoes, halved

a large handful of rocket or other
green salad leaves

salt and freshly ground black pepper

Per serving 4.5g net carbs, 1.6g fibre,
42.4g protein, 27g fat, 428kcal

We love grilling mackerel in the oven or on a barbecue for the speed
of cooking as well as the crispy skin. Use any mustard or even a
combination of grainy and hot English mustards to make the piquant
creamy sauce.

Preheat the grill to hot and grease a roasting tray with a little of the oil.

Make the mustard cream by mixing the mustard, soured cream,
1 teaspoon of lemon zest and some seasoning together in a small bowl.
Taste and adjust the flavourings to taste. Cut the lemon into wedges.

Season the mackerel on both sides and lay on to a baking tray skin-side
up and scatter the tomatoes around it. Season the tomatoes and drizzle
over the remaining oil.

Grill the fish close to the heat source for about 5 minutes or until the skin
is crispy. Depending on the heat of your grill, the mackerel may well be
cooked all the way through. If not, turn it over so that the skin is facing
down and grill for a further couple of minutes.

Serve the fish and tomatoes with the rocket and lemon wedges alongside.

Charlotte's Simple Dahl

SERVES 4 AS A MAIN
(375g/13oz portions) or
6 AS A LIGHTER MEAL
(250g/9oz portions)

1 small onion, finely chopped

a thumb-length piece of fresh ginger,
    peeled and finely chopped or grated

1 garlic clove, finely chopped or grated

2 tablespoons ghee, butter or extra
    virgin olive oil

1 teaspoon smoked paprika

1 teaspoon ground turmeric

2 teaspoons ground cumin

½ teaspoon chilli flakes

320g (11½oz) split red lentils, rinsed

400g (14oz) can cherry or
    plum tomatoes

400g (14oz) can coconut milk

a handful of baby spinach

salt and freshly ground black pepper

a handful of chopped coriander, to serve
    (optional)

Per serving (375g/13oz portion)
11g net carbs, 13.9g fibre, 9.1g
protein, 23.7g fat, 329kcal
Per serving (250g/9oz portion)
7.3g net carbs, 9.3g fibre, 6g protein,
15.8g fat, 219kcal

Charlotte Soin was taught how to make dahl by her Indian grandmother but over the years has added her own twists to the original recipe. This dahl is simple comfort food, but you can also add the odds and ends of chopped vegetables, use it as a base for fried or poached eggs, top it with some crispy fried onions or serve it with a pile of steamed green vegetables doused in chilli oil. For a creamier texture, use a whisk to break up the lentils. I use split red lentils, which are quick to cook and full of insoluble fibre to keep the net carb count down. If you don't have these, use quick-cooking brown ones or cooked and drained green lentils instead.

Fry the onion, ginger and garlic in the ghee for 3 minutes in a medium saucepan. Add the spices, 1 teaspoon of salt and plenty of freshly ground black pepper and stir through, cooking for a minute before stirring in the lentils. Pour in the tomatoes and coconut milk, then fill one of the cans with warm water and add that too. Bring to the boil and as soon as it starts bubbling, reduce the heat and cook for 15–20 minutes or until the lentils are soft. Stir frequently and add a splash more water as necessary to stop the lentils from burning and to achieve a thick, spoonable consistency. Season to taste.

Stir in the spinach and allow it to wilt. Spoon the dahl into warm bowls and serve sprinkled with the coriander, if using.

Beanguine with Pesto & Mozzarella

SERVES 4

700g (1lb 9oz) green beans, such
    as runner or flat beans, or long
    French beans

12 cherry tomatoes (optional)

250g (9oz) mozzarella, drained

For the pesto

15g (½oz) basil leaves, large
    stalks discarded

15g (½oz) Parmesan cheese,
    finely grated

1 small garlic clove

100ml (3½fl oz) extra virgin olive oil

25g (1oz) pine nuts or almonds

salt and freshly ground black pepper

Per serving 10.3g net carbs, 6g fibre,
21.2g protein, 44.2g fat, 525kcal

Green beans make the perfect low-carb swap for pasta in any dish. Buy ready-shredded runner beans if you're feeling lazy, use a bean-slicer for whole runner or flat beans, or simply buy long French beans that only need their stalk ends removed. You can also use frozen beans for this recipe. Like the Italians, I prefer beans soft and flexible rather than firm and squeaky – we are mimicking pasta here – but do cook them to your liking.

Cook the beans in boiling salted water for 5–10 minutes until tender.

Meanwhile, make the pesto by whizzing all the ingredients together in a small food processor or use a pestle and mortar. Taste and adjust the seasoning as necessary. Set aside.

Cut the tomatoes in half, if using (I think they look prettier cut around the middle rather than stalk end to bottom). Tear the mozzarella into bite-sized pieces and leave to drain in a colander over a bowl.

When the beans are soft, drain and divide between 4 warm bowls. Pour over the pesto and scatter over the mozzarella and tomatoes. Serve straight away.

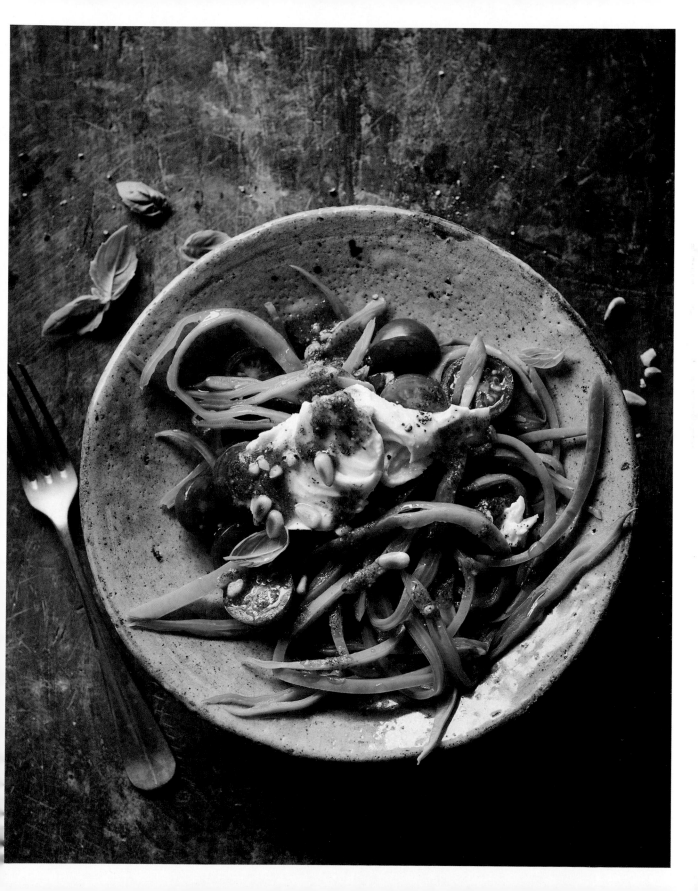

Grilled Paneer & Broccoli Traybake

SERVES 2

1 fat garlic clove, grated

2.5cm (1in) piece of fresh ginger, peeled and grated

5 heaped tablespoons Greek yogurt

1 tablespoon mixed (if you have more than one) curry powder

1 teaspoon hot chilli powder

1 teaspoon ground cumin

1 teaspoon salt

200g (7oz) broccoli, cut into small florets

225g (8oz) paneer, cut into 24 cubes

1 round tomato, weighing about 150g (5½oz), cut into 8 wedges

1 small onion, cut into thin wedges

25g (1oz) butter, melted, or ghee

a small handful of coriander, to serve (optional)

Per serving 14g net carbs, 4.6g fibre, 30g protein, 50g fat, 632kcal

I have kept this simple with broccoli and the Indian cheese paneer, but for more colour you can add red pepper, cauliflower or courgette and serve with coriander or lemon wedges if you want extra prettiness. I have a few different curry powders in my cupboard – I like to buy Indian brands where possible – and enjoy a mix of them with chana masala powder to make up the tablespoon of curry powder used in this recipe. This traybake is a meal on its own, but if you need to stretch it to feed four, then add either Charlotte's Simple Dahl (page 141) or the Cauliflower rice on page 124.

Preheat the grill to hot.

Mix the garlic, ginger, yogurt, spices and salt together in a large mixing bowl. Add the broccoli, paneer, tomato and onion and gently fold into the yogurt mixture.

Spread half the melted butter on to a large baking tray. Spoon over the broccoli and paneer mixture, spreading it out into a single layer. Pour over the remaining butter.

Grill close to the heat for 8–10 minutes, turning once or twice, until the cheese and broccoli are scorched. Scatter with the coriander, if using, and serve straight away.

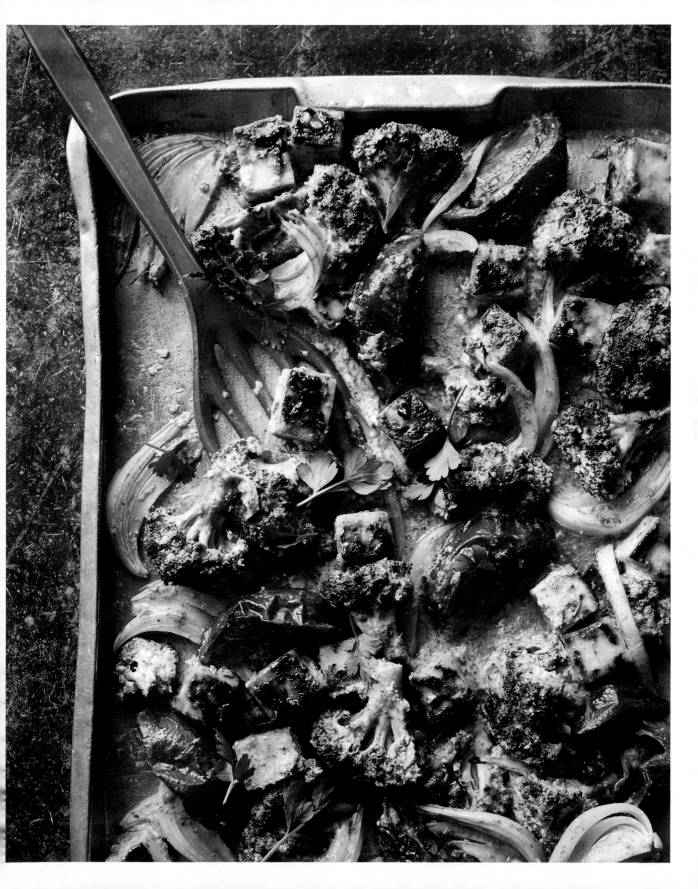

Beetburgers & Avocado Salsa

SERVES 2/MAKES 4 PATTIES

For the beetburgers

olive oil, for greasing

50g (1¾oz) rolled oats

150g (5½oz) raw beetroot, coarsely grated

100g (3½oz) feta cheese, coarsely grated

1 large egg

1 heaped teaspoon ground cumin

salt

For the salsa

2 medium avocados, roughly chopped

200g (7oz) tomatoes, diced

2 teaspoons finely chopped hot green chilli or a pinch of chilli flakes

juice of 1 lime

a few sprigs of coriander or flat-leaf parsley, roughly chopped (optional)

salt and freshly ground black pepper

Per beetburger 10.8g net carbs, 2.3g fibre, 7.3g protein, 7.5g fat, 149kcal
Per serving of avocado salsa 3.6g net carbs, 5.7g fibre, 1.9g protein, 11.6g fat, 137kcal

Beetroot is full of vitamins and minerals and packed with powerful antioxidants. The leaves are good to eat too and even better for you; cook them as you would spinach. The patties are great for lunchboxes and picnics as well as midweek meals.

Preheat the oven to 220°C/200°C fan/425°F/gas mark 7 and lightly grease a baking tray.

To make the beetburgers, whizz the oats in a food processor until they resemble sand. Mix the oats together with the remaining beetburger ingredients in a large bowl, using a large spatula, until well blended. Form the mixture into 4 patties about 8cm (3¼in) wide and 2cm (¾in) deep by squeezing and pressing it together between your palms. They will feel wet but don't worry as it helps to keep them moist during baking. Lay them on to the prepared tray and bake for 20 minutes or until firm the touch and lightly browned.

To make the salsa, gently mix the ingredients together in a bowl and season to taste. Serve the patties warm or at room temperature with the salsa on the side.

Any leftover beetburgers can be wrapped in clingfilm and stored in the fridge for about 3 days.

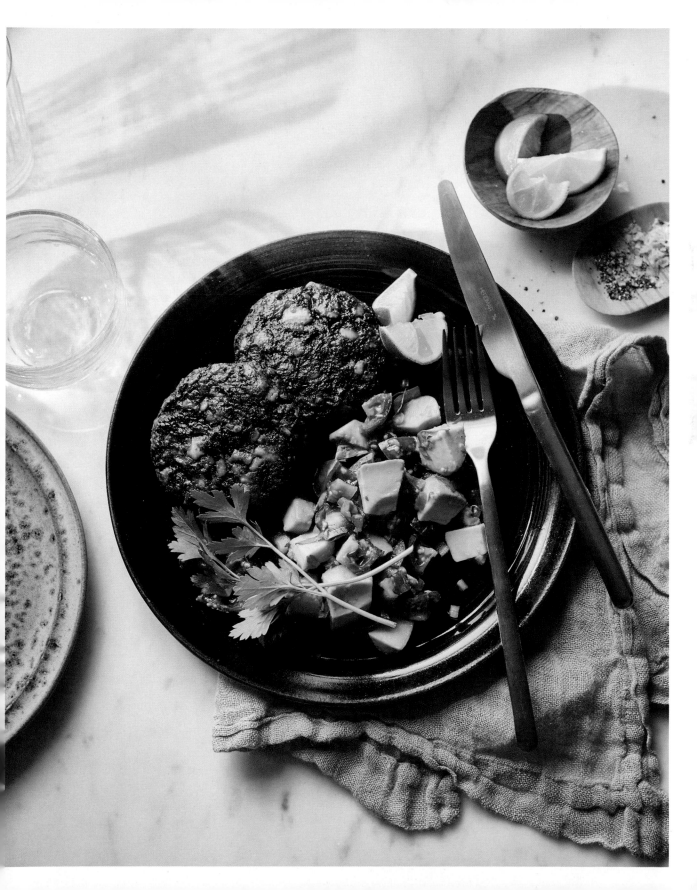

Smoky Aubergines

SERVES 2 AS A MAIN
or 4 AS A SIDE

1 large aubergine, weighing about 400g (14oz)

1 tablespoon extra virgin olive oil

200g (7oz) passata or ½ x 400g (14oz) can chopped tomatoes

½ teaspoon dried oregano

approx. 20 basil leaves

200g (7oz) smoked scamorza, smoked Cheddar cheese or mozzarella, grated

salt and freshly ground black pepper

Per serving 12.4g net carbs, 7.6g fibre, 28.8g protein, 35.9g fat, 499kcal

Smoked scamorza is a wonderful cheese from southern Italy. Similar to firm mozzarella, it can be grated but melts easily. I was so happy to see it make it to the shelves of our local supermarket as it adds such a delicious smoky flavour to dishes, keeps well in the fridge and is so versatile. If you can't find it, use a smoked Cheddar instead. Enjoy the smoky aubergines on their own, with the low-carb bread from page 110 or the green salad on page 57.

Preheat the oven to 240°C/220°C fan/475°F/gas mark 9. Line a baking tray with baking parchment.

Cut the aubergine into circles just under 1cm (½in) thick. Lay them on the prepared tray in a single layer and brush the tops evenly with the oil (you don't need to do the bottoms). Season lightly with salt and pepper. Bake for 10–12 minutes or until golden brown.

Remove the tray from the oven and splash over the passata, then scatter over the oregano and most of the basil leaves followed by the cheese. Return to the oven for 8–10 minutes or until golden brown.

Serve straight away from the tray with the remaining basil scattered over the top.

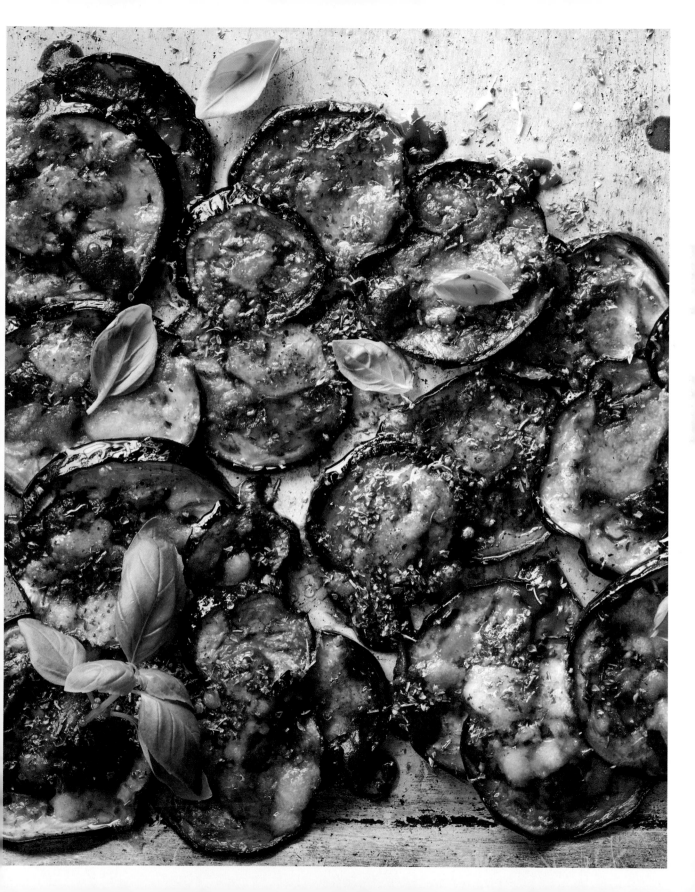

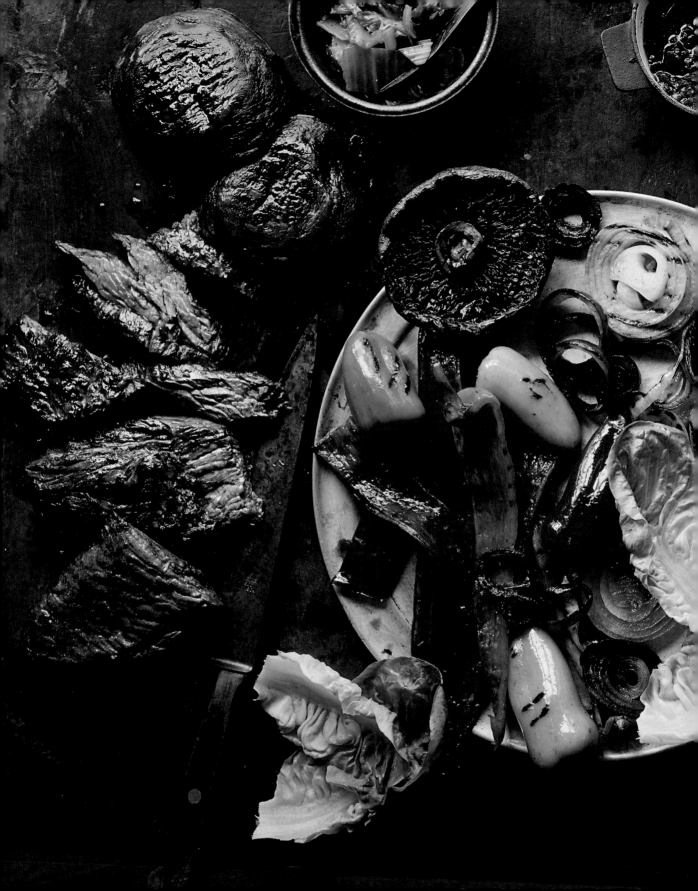

Feeding a *Hungry* Crowd

Lockdown meant we all had to become more inventive with how to feed family and friends, with people enjoying food together in their gardens, on patios and in parks. We dug up our broken fire pit, found an old grill and barbecued on warm, and colder, evenings. We transformed our restaurants into takeaways and provided salads and picnics for people to take to the park. Many of the recipes we created at that time are included here; easy and quick ideas to make feeding family and friends fun and effortless.

Charred Tomatoes, Labneh & Flatbreads

SERVES 6

For the tomatoes

300g (10½oz) cherry tomatoes

1 small onion, cut into 10 wedges

4 tablespoons extra virgin olive oil

1 teaspoon dried oregano

4 garlic cloves in their skins,
  lightly crushed

salt and freshly ground black pepper

For the flatbreads

50g (1¾oz) ground almonds

10g (¼oz) psyllium husk

2 tablespoons coconut flour

1 teaspoon baking powder

1 tablespoon cumin, black onion
  (nigella), sesame or coriander
  seeds (optional)

a knob of ghee, butter or coconut oil

For the labneh

100g (3½oz) feta or goat's cheese

200g (7oz) thick Greek or
  strained yogurt

1 tablespoon extra virgin olive oil

a handful of basil, coriander or flat-leaf
  parsley leaves

Per serving (including flatbread)
6.3g net carbs, 3.8g fibre, 6.7g protein,
25.2g fat, 290kcal

This stunning dish is good enough for a meal on its own or can be prepared for a buffet or as part of a barbecue. The flatbreads complement almost any dish and keep well for a day or two in the fridge in an airtight container. You can enjoy them plain, or add cumin, black onion (nigella), sesame or coriander seeds. I like a slick of ghee, butter or olive oil over the top too.

When you have made the bread once, you will know the pan and correct heat to use. On my hob, 9 is the maximum heat and about 7.5 does the job. Too hot and the bread burns before cooking inside, too low and they take ages to cook and you don't get the characteristic scorch marks of bread cooked in a tandoor oven.

Preheat the oven to 220°C/200°C fan/475°F/gas mark 7.

Put all the ingredients for the tomatoes in an ovenproof dish, season and toss to combine. Cook for 18–20 minutes.

Meanwhile, make the flatbreads. Mix the dry ingredients and ½ teaspoon of salt together in a bowl and add 150ml (5fl oz) water. Use your hands to mix it into a dough, then set aside for 5 minutes to allow the water to be absorbed. Divide the dough into 12 and roll each piece into a ball.

Heat a non-stick frying pan over a medium-high heat. Roll one ball of dough between two pieces of baking parchment to a thickness of about 3mm (⅛in); don't worry about the raggedy edges. Add a knob of ghee to the pan and swirl the pan so it coats the base – you only need a light covering. (If your pan is very non-stick, you may not need any ghee or oil.)

Peel the flatbread off the parchment and lay in the pan. Cook for 3 minutes on each side, depending on the heat, until well browned and cooked through. Roll the next flatbread as the first cooks, then add to the pan. Repeat with the remaining dough. You can use a spatula to flip the flatbreads and hold them down if they puff up.

As the last flatbread cooks, prepare the labneh by mashing the cheese, yogurt and oil together with a fork. Spread the labneh on to a plate.

Pour the tomatoes and their cooking oil, over the labneh, then scatter over the herbs. Serve straight away with the flatbreads on the side.

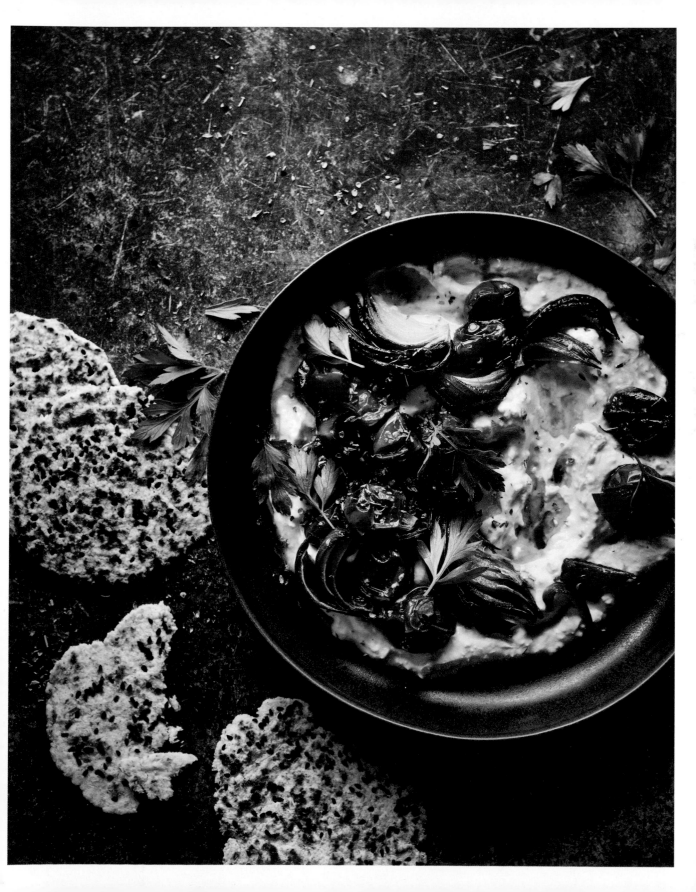

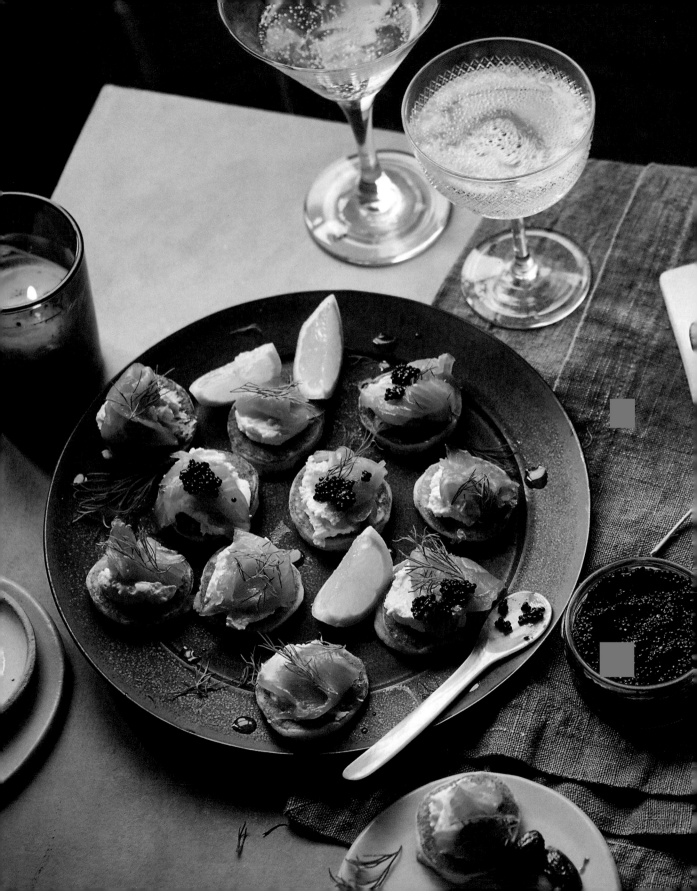

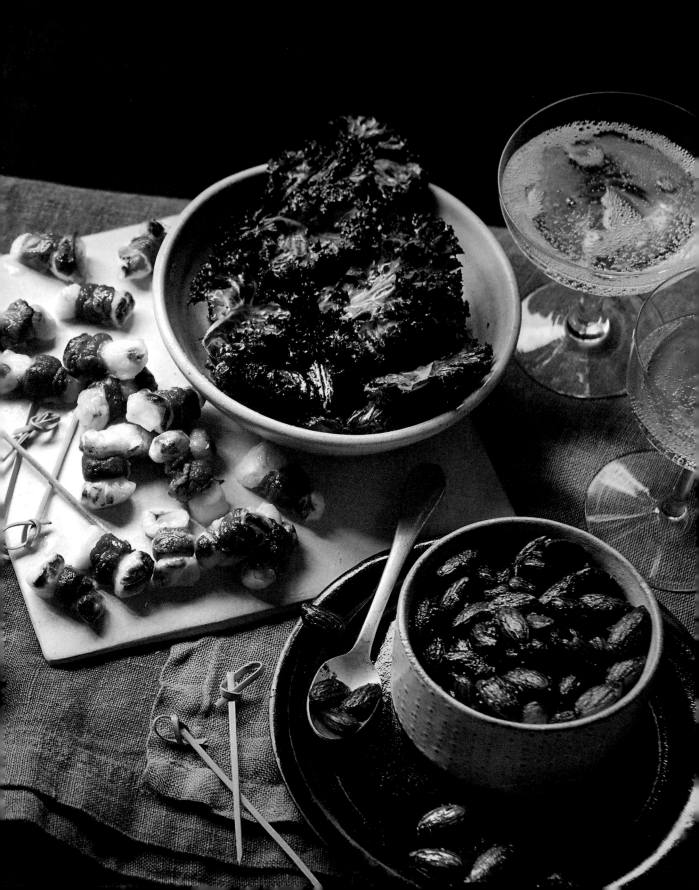

Easy Blinis

SERVES 10/ MAKES APPROX. 40
SMALL (4CM) BLINIS

2 tablespoons coconut flour

1 teaspoon baking powder

50g (1¾oz) ground almonds

¼ teaspoon salt

2 eggs

1 tablespoon butter, melted

100ml (3½fl oz) whole or almond milk

a little coconut oil, ghee or dripping

Topping ideas

butter, cheese and a torn celery leaf

cream cheese, salmon or caviar

smashed avocado, lemon and chilli

Per serving of 4 blinis 1.5g net carbs,
1g fibre, 2.6g protein, 5.2g fat, 67kcal

This recipe works for savoury and sweet blinis and has enough body to carry a topping. They keep well in the fridge for 3 days, make a quick breakfast and can be turned into a snack or starter.

Whisk the coconut flour, baking powder, ground almonds and salt together in a mixing bowl. Add the eggs and stir through briefly before adding the melted butter. Stir in the milk, a little at a time, until you have a smooth batter; if your eggs are large you may need less.

If you have a good non-stick pan you probably won't need any fat to cook the blinis. If not, melt a knob of fat in a large frying pan with a flat base (or use a crêpe pan) over a medium-high heat and swirl to coat the base of the pan. Use a dessertspoon to drop half a spoonful of batter into the pan. It should spread into a circle, but you can use the spoon to nudge it into shape. Let it bubble and become lightly brown around the edges. When it is set enough to turn, use a thin slice to flip it over. Let it brown again for a minute and once it has lost its wobble, transfer to a wooden board. Taste and adjust the salt and consistency as you like.

Cook the remaining batter, working clockwise around the pan so you know which blini has to be turned first. Add a drop more fat if they begin to stick. Enjoy straight away or leave to cool depending on your topping.

Spicy Almonds

SERVES 10

200g (7oz) almonds

2 tablespoon extra virgin olive oil

2 teaspoons dried oregano

2 teaspoons sweet paprika

¾–1 teaspoon salt

½–1 teaspoon hot chilli powder or
cayenne pepper

Per 20g serving 1.8g net carbs, 2.5g
fibre, 4.2g protein, 12.7g fat, 139kcal

If you don't have almonds, you can use pecans, walnuts or macadamia but they have different cooking times, so watch them like a hawk.

Preheat the oven to 220°C/200°C fan/475°F/gas mark 7 and line an oven tray with baking parchment.

Toss the almonds with the remaining ingredients, adding the chilli powder to taste. Transfer to the prepared tray and cook for 6 minutes or until golden brown. Remove from the oven and slide the parchment on to a cool work surface so the nuts stop cooking straight away. When warm or cool, as you prefer, use the parchment to shoot them into a bowl and serve. They will keep well in an airtight container for up to 3 days.

Cheesy Garlicky Kale Crisps

SERVES 6

200g (7oz) kale, ribs removed

2 teaspoons smoked paprika

½ teaspoon salt

2 heaped teaspoons black onion (nigella) seeds

2 tablespoons extra virgin olive oil

2 heaped teaspoons garlic powder

2 tablespoons finely grated Parmesan or Grana Padano cheese

freshly ground black pepper

Per serving 1.1g net carbs, 1.4g fibre, 1.7g protein, 5.5g fat, 64kcal

Use any firm green leaves from the cabbage family, such as kale, cauliflower or even Brussels sprouts for these crisps. Don't wash the leaves unless they are muddy, in which case shake them well and dry them on kitchen paper.

Preheat the oven to 220°C/200°C fan/475°F/gas mark 7.

Roughly tear the kale leaves into bite-sized pieces – the same size as large potato crisps. Put these in a bowl with the remaining ingredients and mix together using your hands or a large spoon. Spread them over a large oven tray in a single layer. You may need two trays.

Cook for 5 minutes or until crisp and light. Serve straight away or leave to cool. Any leftovers will keep for a couple of days in an airtight container. If they become soft, put them back in a hot oven for a couple of minutes to firm up again.

Halloumi & Bacon Bites

SERVES 12

16 rashers of smoked streaky bacon

225g (8oz) halloumi, cut into 36 small pieces

Per serving of 3 bites 0.3g net carbs, 0g fibre, 6.5g protein, 9.6g fat, 114kcal

These can be knocked up quickly, particularly if one person preps the bacon and the other rolls up the bites. Any leftovers are lovely chopped into a salad or soup.

Preheat the oven to 220°C/200°C fan/475°F/gas mark 7. Line a baking tray with baking parchment.

If the bacon is very thin, leave it as it is. If not, lay the rashers on a chopping board and scrape a cook's knife over them at an angle to stretch them out. Cut into 36 pieces.

Put a piece of halloumi on one end of each rasher and roll them up. Transfer to the baking tray and cook for 10–12 minutes or until the bacon is cooked through. Transfer to a serving dish and serve them just as they are cool enough to handle.

Whipped Chicken Liver Pâté

SERVES 10

125g (4½oz) butter, softened

1 onion, finely sliced into half-moons

*2 teaspoons thyme leaves,
  finely chopped*

*400g (14oz) chicken livers,
  roughly chopped*

*4 tablespoons Cognac, brandy or
  white wine*

5 tablespoons double cream

½ teaspoon ground nutmeg

½ teaspoon ground cinnamon

salt and freshly ground black pepper

Per serving 1.4g net carbs, 0.1g fibre,
10.1g protein, 16.3g fat, 208kcal

This has dish has recently become fashionable in New York, which is great news as we should all be eating more offal. Liver is packed with nutrients, inexpensive and quick to cook. This über-healthy dish is so good it will persuade even the most committed offal-hater. You usually have to get rid of the white connective tissue when cooking chicken livers, but since the pâté is blitzed until smooth you don't need to bother, making this even easier to cook. I like to serve the pâté in a bowl on a wooden chopping board, topped with caramelized onions and thyme. I put a couple of knives around it and a few Focaccia Sticks or slices of toasted Bap (page 110) and let everyone dig in.

Melt 25g (1oz) of the butter in a frying pan over a medium heat, add the onion and half the thyme and fry for about 7 minutes or until the onion has softened. Tip half the mixture on to a plate and set aside. Add the livers to the pan and cook for about 4 minutes or until firm when squeezed, browned on the outside but still pale pink inside.

Add the Cognac, bring to the boil over a high heat and bubble for 2 minutes. Tip the mixture into a high-speed food processor, add the cream, nutmeg, cinnamon and ½ teaspoon of salt and blitz until smooth. Add the remaining butter in three stages, blitzing between each one until smooth. Taste and adjust the seasoning as necessary using plenty of freshly ground black pepper. Transfer to a serving bowl and top with the reserved onion and thyme.

Serve the pâté warm or leave to cool to room temperature and accompany with low-carb baps or focaccia sticks (page 110), raw pepper slices, lettuce or chicory leaves. Once cooled the pâté will keep in an airtight container in the fridge for up to 3 days.

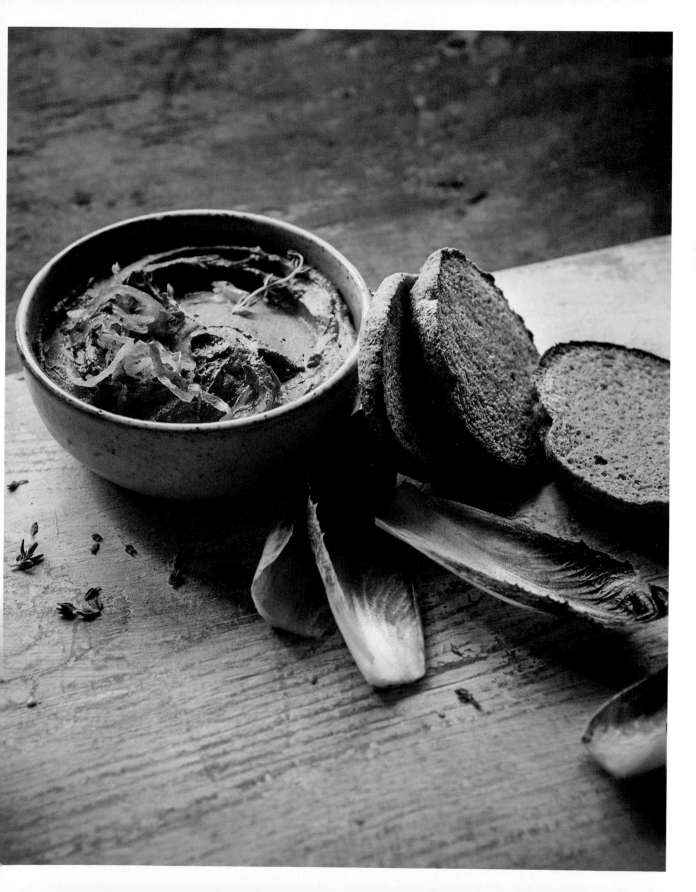

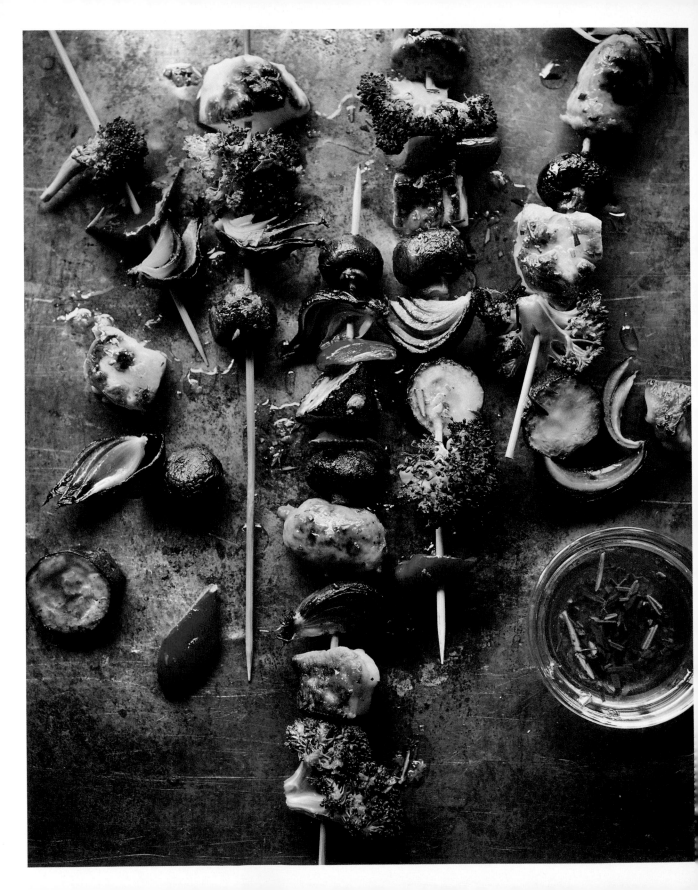

Sausage & Halloumi Kebabs or Traybake

SERVES 6

500g (1lb 2oz) mixture of courgettes, mushrooms, peppers and/or broccoli

1 red or brown onion, cut into thick wedges

225g (8oz) halloumi, cut into 2cm (¾in) cubes

6 sausages, weighing about 275g (9¾oz), each one cut into 3

2 tablespoons extra virgin olive oil

salad leaves, to serve

For the dressing

3 tablespoons extra virgin olive oil

zest and juice of ½ lemon

1 sprig of rosemary, leaves finely chopped

salt and freshly ground black pepper

Per serving 6.4g net carbs, 3g fibre, 18.8g protein, 34g fat, 412kcal

This is lovely in summer cooked over a fire or under the grill in cooler months. It uses up vegetables from the fridge and it's a real crowd-pleaser. If time allows or you have a friendly sous chef, make up the skewers by alternating the ingredients between them. If time is short and you are on your own, put the ingredients on to a large baking tray. You don't even need to cut the sausages.

Preheat your indoor grill to high or light the barbecue.

Cut the courgettes into 2cm (¾in) slices, halve the mushrooms, dice the pepper into 3cm (1¼in) pieces and cut the broccoli into bite-sized florets. Separate the onion wedges into double layers.

To make the kebabs, alternate the vegetables, cheese and sausages on to metal skewers (if you are using wooden skewers do soak them in water for at least 10 minutes first). Drizzle over the oil and season, turning them to ensure an even covering.

To make the traybake, toss the vegetables, halloumi and sausages on a large oven tray with the oil and seasoning and spread out in a single layer; make sure all the vegetables have a little oil and seasoning and that there aren't dry, unloved ones sitting in the corners.

Cook the kebabs over a barbecue or the traybake under the hot grill for 8–10 minutes, turning a couple of times or until the sausages are cooked through.

To make the dressing, stir all the ingredients together in a jug.

Serve the kebabs and salad leaves on a wooden board with a rim to catch the juices or serve the traybake in the oven tray or transfer to a serving dish, putting the salad leaves in a bowl on the side. Eat straight away and let everyone pour the dressing on to their plates.

30-minute Korean Barbecue

SERVES 6

3 medium onions

6 medium portobello mushrooms

2 red bell or Romano peppers

4 ribeye or sirloin steaks, or 1 bavette
  steak or 1kg (2lb 4oz) pork belly,
  thinly sliced

3 Little Gem or 1–2 Romaine lettuces

2 tablespoons toasted sesame seeds,
  to serve

kimchi, to serve (optional)

For the sauce

4 tablespoons tamari or dark soy sauce

1 tablespoon toasted sesame oil

2 garlic cloves, finely chopped

1 shallot or small onion or 5 spring
  onions, finely chopped

1 red-hot Thai chilli, finely chopped, to
  taste, or ½ teaspoon chilli flakes

approx. 15g (½oz) fresh ginger, peeled
  and grated

2 teaspoons honey

3 tablespoons sake, sherry or water

Per serving with steak 15g net carbs,
8.2g fibre, 40.4g protein, 23.7g fat,
452kcal
Per serving with pork belly 12.3g net
carbs, 5.8g fibre, 38.4g protein, 38g
fat, 556kcal

In the time it takes to get the fire ready, you can prepare the sauce and vegetables for this delicious Korean-inspired barbecue. If you don't fancy finding your inner caveman, you can just grill or pan-fry the steaks instead. To make this truly Korean, use a meat mallet to bash the steaks to a thickness of about 5mm (¼in) and cut them into seven 5cm (2¾ x 2in) rectangles. However, cooking the steaks whole and then slicing them gives a wonderful result in much less time. Inexpensive bavette steak or thinly sliced pork belly also work well.

Light the barbecue.

Put all the sauce ingredients plus 125ml (4fl oz) water in a frying pan and bring to the boil. Reduce the heat and simmer for about 5 minutes until the sauce has reduced by a third. Unless you are exceptionally good at chopping and your pieces of onion and ginger are small, blitz the sauce briefly in a food processor. Transfer the sauce to a jug and put it on a large chopping board with a rim to catch the meat juices.

Meanwhile, cut the onions into rings just under 1cm (½in) thick, keeping them intact so that they don't fall through the grill. Remove the stalks from the mushrooms and slice each bell pepper into 6 long strips or each Romano pepper into 4 long strips. When the coals are ready, cook the onions, mushrooms and peppers for about 5 minutes on each side until tender and lightly browned. Set aside in a warm place.

Lay the meat of your choice on the grill. There is no need to season the meat as the sauce is salty enough. Depending on how hot your grill is, and how close it is to the source of heat, cook the steaks for a few minutes on each side until done to your liking, then set aside to rest. As a rough guide, cook a fingerwidth steak for 2 minutes each side for rare, 2–3 minutes each side for medium rare and 4 minutes each side for well done. Bavette usually needs 4 minutes a side and the pork belly slices just a couple of minutes a side.

Separate the lettuce leaves and add these and the barbecued vegetables to the serving board in piles. Serve the kimchi in a bowl, if using. Slice the steaks and lay on to the board. Pour a little of the sauce over each one and scatter over the sesame seeds. Serve straight away; use the lettuce leaves as containers for the cut steak and vegetables and drizzle over a little more sauce.

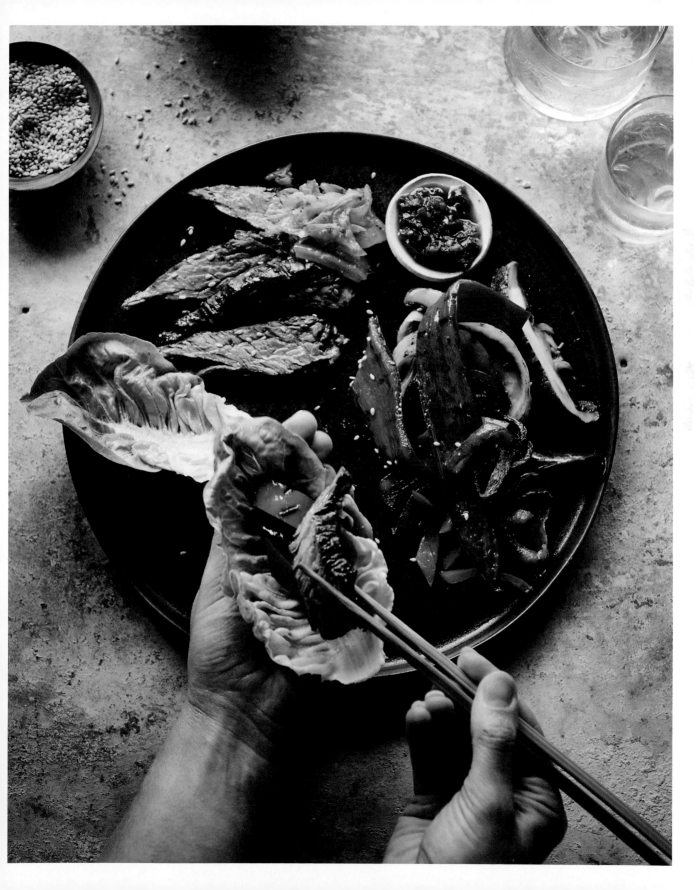

Chicken & Chilli Sauce

SERVES 6

2 tablespoons extra virgin olive oil

3 rosemary sprigs, halved

12 boneless and skinless chicken thighs

2 onions, cut into 8 wedges

2 red bell or Romano peppers

2 courgettes or 1 aubergine or
   1 small head of broccoli

2 handfuls of watercress, rocket
   or lettuce

salt and freshly ground black pepper

1 lemon, cut into wedges, to serve

For the chilli sauce

1–2 red chillies, depending on strength,
   or ½ teaspoon chilli flakes

2 garlic cloves

6 tablespoons olive oil

1 sprig of rosemary, stem discarded

¼ teaspoon salt and plenty of freshly
   ground black pepper

Per serving 5.2g net carbs, 1.9g fibre,
40.7g protein, 26.8g fat, 439kcal

This simple traybake can be easily adapted to whatever vegetables you have in the fridge that roast well, such as peppers, courgettes, aubergines, tomatoes or broccoli. For a slightly more adventurous version, try fennel bulbs, pumpkin or radicchio. I've allowed two chicken thighs per person as supermarket ones tend to be small. If I buy chicken thighs from my butcher, they are huge and one per person is plenty, so the choice is yours.

Preheat the oven to 220°C/200°C fan/475°F/gas mark 7.

Lightly oil a baking tray with 1 teaspoon of the oil and scatter over the rosemary. Season the chicken thighs on both sides and lay them over the rosemary, stretching them out flat so that they cook quickly. Scatter the onions, peppers and courgettes around the edges of the chicken, season and drizzle with the remaining oil. Cook for 20–25 minutes until the chicken thighs are cooked through. There should be no pink juices when you pierce the thickest part of the thigh or the internal temperature should be higher than 74°C (165°F).

Meanwhile, make the sauce. Taste one of the red chillies from the middle of the chilli where the pith joins the seeds to see how hot they are and decide whether one or two will do the job. If neither are spicy enough, add a pinch of chilli flakes. Put all the sauce ingredients in a small food processor and whizz to combine or chop finely by hand and mix together. Transfer to a jug and set aside.

Divide the cooked chicken and vegetables between 6 plates. Add a little watercress and a lemon wedge to each plate and serve with the sauce on the side.

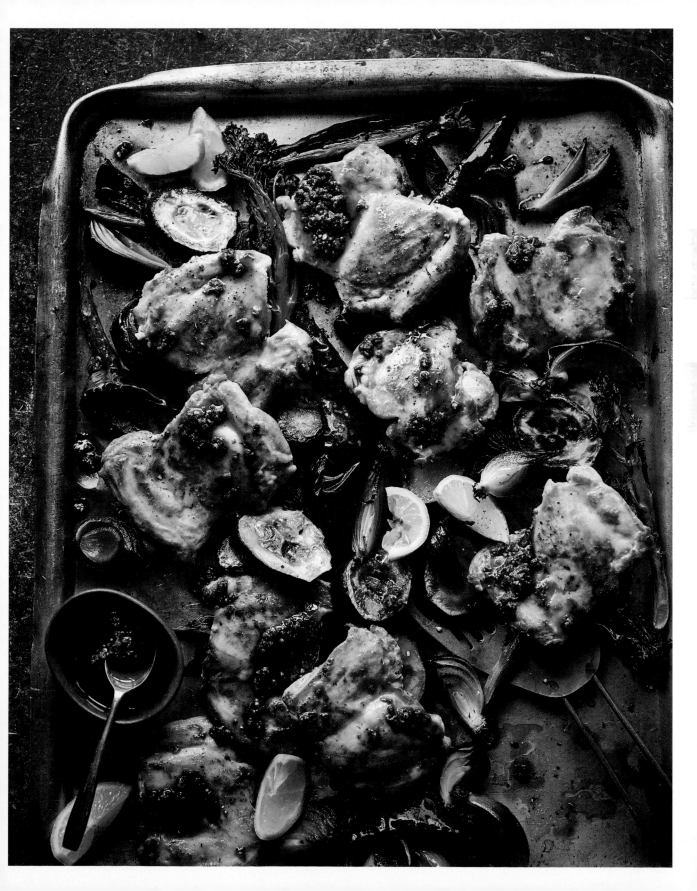

Herby Fishcakes with Courgette Salad

SERVES 4/MAKES 8 FISHCAKES

approx. 520g (1lb 3oz) white fish fillets,
* such as haddock, cod or coley*

1 medium onion, roughly chopped

10g (¼oz) mint leaves

10g (¼oz) coriander or flat-leaf parsley,
* stalks and leaves roughly chopped*

2 tablespoons extra virgin olive oil, ghee
* or coconut oil*

For the courgette salad

2 medium courgettes, weighing about
* 275g (9¾oz)*

2 tablespoons extra virgin olive oil

juice of ½ lemon

1 mild red chilli, finely sliced, or a pinch
* of chilli flakes*

1 garlic clove, grated

salt and freshly ground black pepper

Per serving of 2 fishcakes 4g net
carbs, 1g fibre, 25.6g protein, 15.5g
fat, 268kcal

These fishcakes are so quick to prepare. Any white fish is suitable, such as haddock, cod or coley. When I'm catering for a crowd, I buy bags of frozen white fish and defrost them overnight. The courgette salad recipe is from our good friend Inna Skachko, who rustles it up frequently at our house as I always have courgettes in the fridge. She makes the salad while I prepare the fishcakes and food is on the table in less than 30 minutes. This makes a light meal; to bump it up with healthy fats, add some sliced avocado to the salad or serve the fishcakes in the low-carb Baps on page 110.

Cut the fish fillets into 3 pieces and pop them into a food processor, squeezing out any juices if the fish was frozen. Add the onion, herbs and 1 teaspoon of salt and whizz to form a rough paste. Divide the mixture into 8 and use your hands to form even-sized fishcakes.

Fry the fishcakes in the oil over a medium-high heat for about 4 minutes on each side or until lightly browned and cooked through.

Meanwhile, make the salad. Slice the courgettes with a vegetable peeler. Add the remaining ingredients and stir through. Taste and adjust the seasoning and serve with the fishcakes.

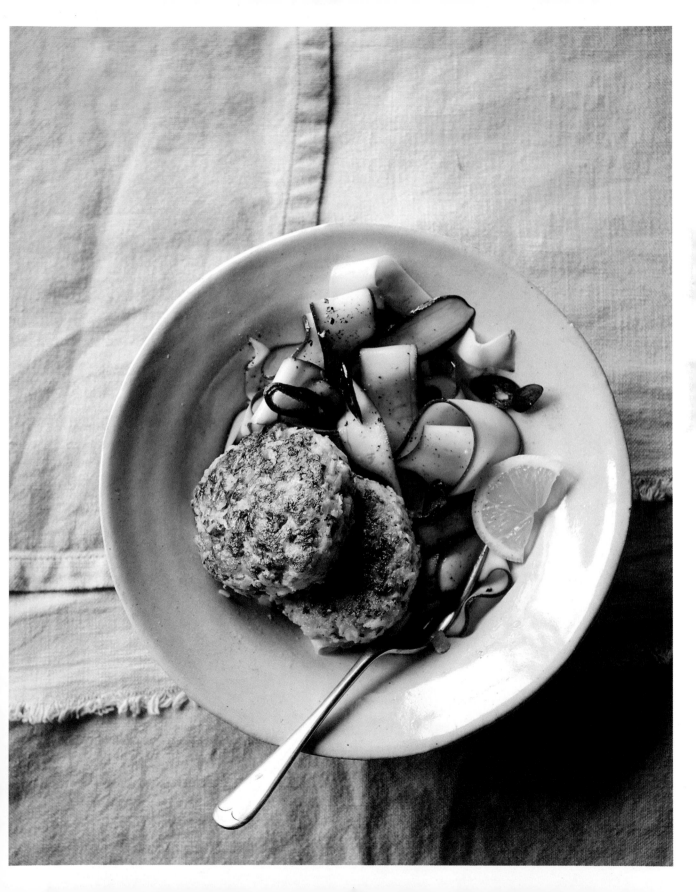

Pizza Pronto

MAKES 1 TRAY PIZZA APPROX. 35 X 30CM (14 X 12IN)/SERVES 6

For the pizza base

1 quantity of Quick Brown Bread dough (page 110)

For the tomato sauce

100g (3½oz) tomato passata or puréed canned tomatoes

½ teaspoon dried oregano

¼ teaspoon salt

1 tablespoon extra virgin olive oil

Topping ideas (optional)

125g (4½oz) mozzarella ball, drained

12 black or green olives, stoned

6 slices of salami

25g (1oz) mushrooms, sliced

1 red or green chilli, finely sliced or chilli flakes, to taste

1 tablespoon extra virgin olive oil

To serve (optional)

tomatoes, chopped

a handful of basil leaves

a small handful of rocket leaves

6 slices of prosciutto

Per serving (with 3 slices of salami and 3 slices of prosciutto) 5.9g net carbs, 9.9g fibre, 16.7g protein, 31.3g fat, 410kcal

This quick dough is easier to make than traditional wheat dough; there is no rising time and the base is a fraction of the carbs of a traditional pizza. Topping ideas are endless but I have given a few suggestions below. Don't be tempted by the ready-grated mozzarella, some brands contain potato starch making it higher in carbs and it takes longer to melt. Serve the pizza as it is or with a crisp green salad, see page 57.

Preheat the oven to 240°C/220°C fan/475°F/gas mark 9. Line a 35 × 30cm (14 × 12in) baking tray with baking parchment.

Follow the instructions for making the dough on page 110 and put it on to the lined tray. With wet hands, press and shape the dough into a rectangle just less than a 1cm (½in) deep to fill the tray. Bake for 8 minutes or until it feels firm to the touch.

Meanwhile, stir the tomato sauce ingredients together in a small bowl.

Remove the tray from the oven. Pour the sauce over the base and spread it out using a spoon or leave some areas without it. Add the toppings of your choice and drizzle over the olive oil. I have separated the topping ideas that can be cooked and "to serve" topping suggestions that are better added after cooking. In the photo on the cover, I cooked half the pizza with salami and added prosciutto after cooking to the remaining half as we like the variation.

Bake for 7 minutes or until the mozzarella is bubbling and the crust is crisp and brown. Remove from the oven and top the with fresh basil, rocket and prosciutto, if using. Cut into 6 slices and serve straight away.

Hülya's Aubergines

SERVES 6

1 medium aubergine

1 courgette

1 onion

1 red pepper

4 tablespoons extra virgin olive oil

2 garlic cloves, crushed

½ teaspoon chilli flakes (optional)

400g (14oz) can chopped tomatoes or 400g (14oz) passata

1 tablespoon red wine or other vinegar

6 tablespoons Greek yogurt (optional)

salt and freshly ground black pepper

Per serving 10.7g net carbs, 3.8g fibre, 2.5g protein, 9.9g fat, 150kcal

This is a really useful Turkish dish made by our friend Hülya Kocu. She cooks enough to have some left over for a few days in the fridge and uses it as a base for various toppings. She adds crumbled feta and coriander or parsley one day, fried eggs another or grilled lamb cutlets the next day. Don't worry if you don't have all the vegetables; just use more of one you do have. If you like it spicy, add a good pinch of chilli flakes or a teaspoon or two of harissa paste.

Cut the vegetables into bite-sized pieces.

Pour the oil into a large frying pan or wok over a high heat, add the vegetables, garlic and chilli, if using, season and stir-fry for 10 minutes.

Add the tomatoes and vinegar and bring to the boil. Reduce the heat to medium and cook for a further 5–10 minutes to thicken. Taste and add further seasoning as necessary.

Serve with the yogurt, if using.

Topping suggestions

25g (1oz) feta cheese, crumbled per person

a small handful of coriander or flat-leaf parsley, leaves roughly chopped and stems finely chopped per person

2 fried or poached eggs per person

2 small lamb cutlets per person

Israeli Sabich Salad with Feta

SERVES 6

800g (1lb 12oz) aubergines

5 tablespoons extra virgin olive oil

6 eggs

1 long cucumber

3 large, firm tomatoes

5 spring onions (optional)

juice of 1 lemon

2 tablespoons harissa paste

2 tablespoons tahini

2 teaspoons amba (optional)

100g (3½oz) feta cheese, crumbled

2 tablespoons coriander or flat-leaf parsley leaves

salt and freshly ground black pepper

Per serving 13.8g net carbs, 5.2g fibre, 11g protein, 23g fat, 312kcal

Sabich is an Israeli vegetarian dish introduced to me by private chef Fabienne Viner Luzzata. It's normally stuffed into a pitta bread, which spoils its beauty and whacks up the carbs. Fabienne showed me her way of making it as a stunning salad, perfect for a light lunch or supper. She uses amba, a strong-flavoured sauce made from pickled green mangoes, to finish the dish. It's not essential, but it is a delicious addition, and can be bought from delis or online and used as a condiment for roast meats, eggs or the Cauliflower Couscous on page 124. To make this vegan, omit the eggs and use chickpeas instead of the feta.

Preheat the oven to 220°C/200°C fan/425°F/gas mark 7 and line 1–2 baking trays with baking parchment.

Slice the aubergines into circles just less than 1cm (½in) thick. Lay them on the prepared trays and brush the tops with 2 tablespoons of the oil. Season and cook for 15–18 minutes or until lightly browned. Remove from the oven tray and set aside to cool.

Meanwhile, cook the eggs. Bring a large saucepan of water to the boil, add the eggs and cook for 6 minutes exactly. Remove the eggs from the water with a slotted spoon and plunge them into cold water, then crack the shells to avoid a blue circle forming around the yolk. Peel them when cool enough to handle.

Peel the cucumber and cut into four lengthwise. Finely chop the cucumber strips and the tomatoes, then cut the spring onions into small slices, if using. Mix them together in a bowl with 2 tablespoons of the olive oil, the lemon juice and some seasoning, and spread the mixture out on a large serving dish.

Lay the cooked aubergines over the top of the salad and spread each one with a little harissa. Drizzle over the tahini (if it's very thick, add a little cold water to dilute it). Slice the eggs and lay pieces over the aubergines. If you are using the amba, spread just a little over the eggs here and there with a knife. Season the eggs with a little salt and pepper. Drizzle over the remaining tablespoon of oil, scatter over the feta and herbs and you are ready to serve.

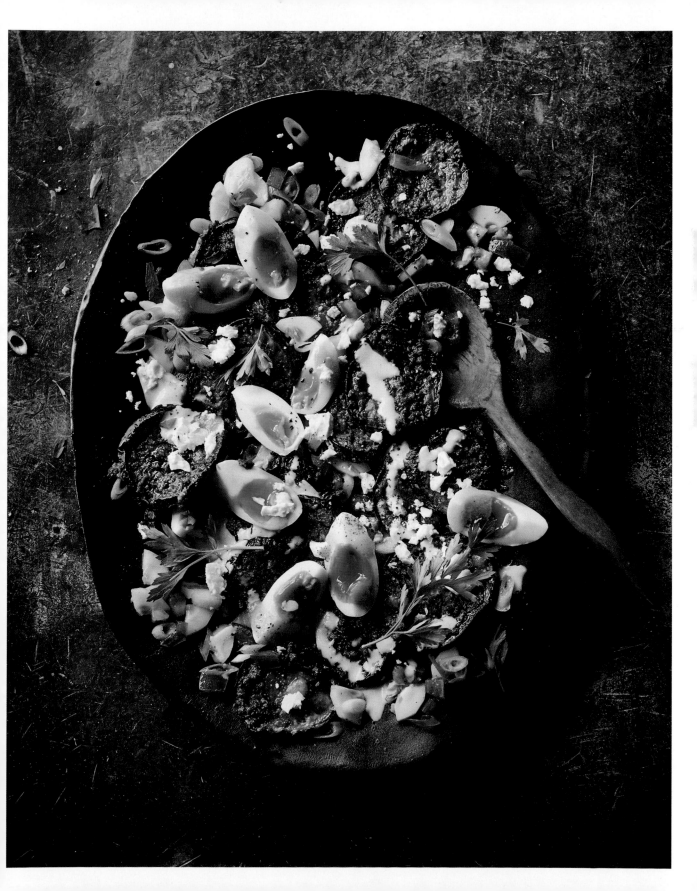

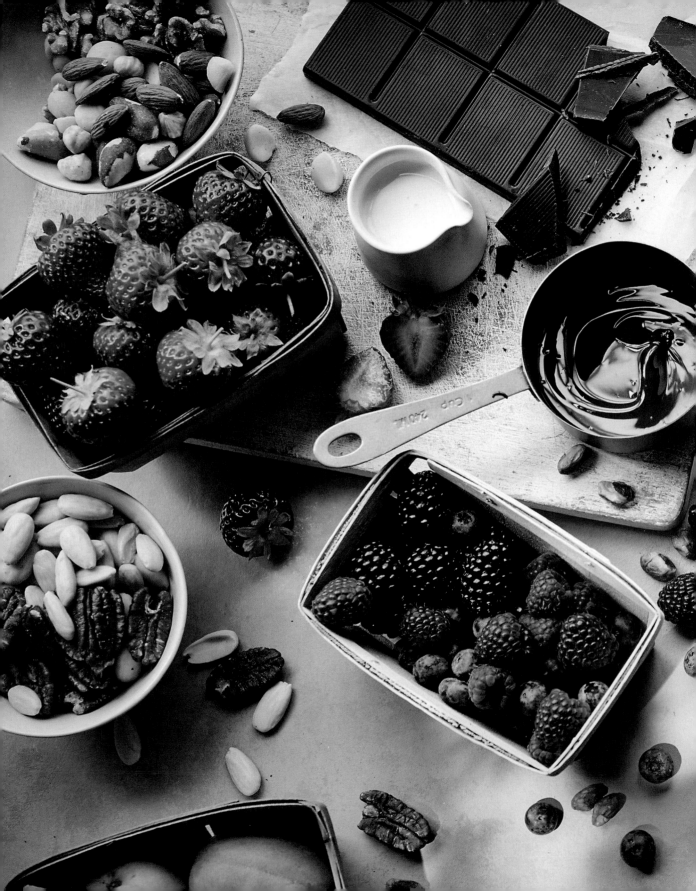

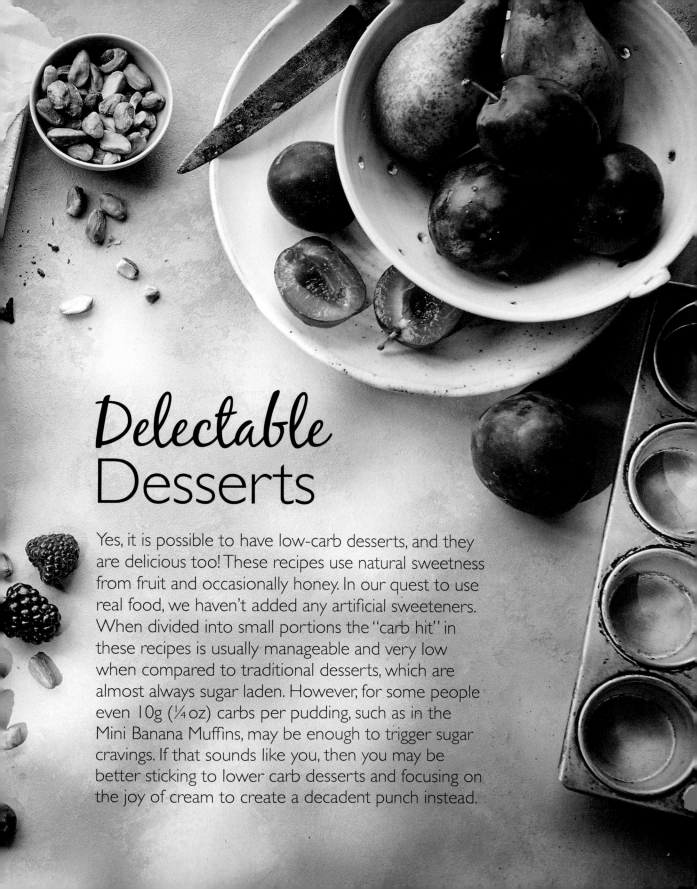

Delectable
Desserts

Yes, it is possible to have low-carb desserts, and they are delicious too! These recipes use natural sweetness from fruit and occasionally honey. In our quest to use real food, we haven't added any artificial sweeteners. When divided into small portions the "carb hit" in these recipes is usually manageable and very low when compared to traditional desserts, which are almost always sugar laden. However, for some people even 10g (¼oz) carbs per pudding, such as in the Mini Banana Muffins, may be enough to trigger sugar cravings. If that sounds like you, then you may be better sticking to lower carb desserts and focusing on the joy of cream to create a decadent punch instead.

Blueberry & Lemon Ice Cream

SERVES 6

250g (9oz) mascarpone

zest of 1 lemon

150g (5½oz) frozen blueberries

1 teaspoon honey (optional)

Per serving 5g net carbs, 0.6g fibre, 1.5g protein, 19g fat, 194kcal

This instant ice cream is perfect for whipping up on a hot summer's day. It can be made with other frozen berries, such as strawberries or raspberries, or a mixture of all three.

Put 6 small glasses or espresso cups in the fridge or freezer to chill.

Whizz all the ingredients together in a food processor until just smooth. Don't overmix or it will melt. Spoon into the chilled glasses and serve straight away.

If it does melt, serve anyway and just tell people it is a smoothie; it is still delicious!

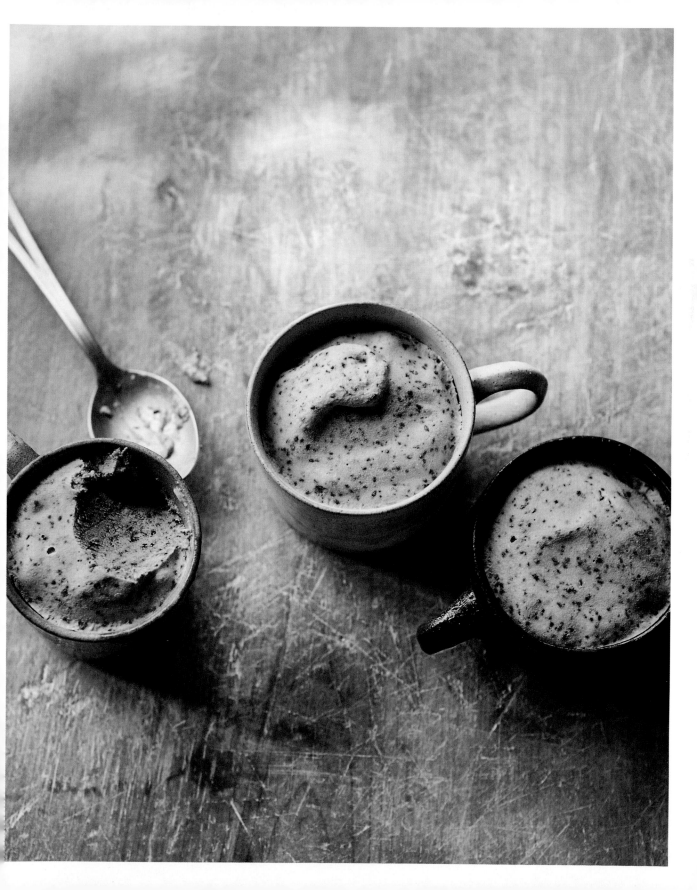

Baked Cheesecakes with Summer Berries

SERVES 6

450g (1lb) cream cheese

150g (5½oz) soured cream

2 eggs

2 teaspoons vanilla extract

200g (7oz) mixed berries, such as raspberries, blackberries, blueberries or strawberries, hulled and quartered if large

Per serving 9.6g net carbs, 1g fibre, 8g protein, 30.3g fat, 304kcal

Stefano Borella is the patisserie chef at our restaurant Caldesi in Marylebone in London. Over the years I have convinced him to cut back on sugar, and then he surprised me with this no-sugar version of his famous cheesecake. It's delicious and, by using vanilla, it doesn't need any sugar at all. Eat the cheesecakes still warm or enjoy them chilled from the fridge. Top with berries, such as raspberries, blackberries, blueberries or strawberries, or any seasonal low-carb fruit. If you don't have ramekins, small tea or coffee cups do the trick and they don't have to match.

Preheat the oven to 220°C/200°C fan/425°F/gas mark 7.

Whisk the cream cheese, soured cream, eggs and vanilla together in a mixing bowl and spoon into 6 ramekins. If you want to be precise you should have around 120ml (4fl oz) for each portion.

Put the cheesecakes on to a baking tray and cook for 15–17 minutes or until just firm to the touch. They will set firm on cooling.

Top with the berries just before serving. Any leftovers will keep for 2 days in the fridge.

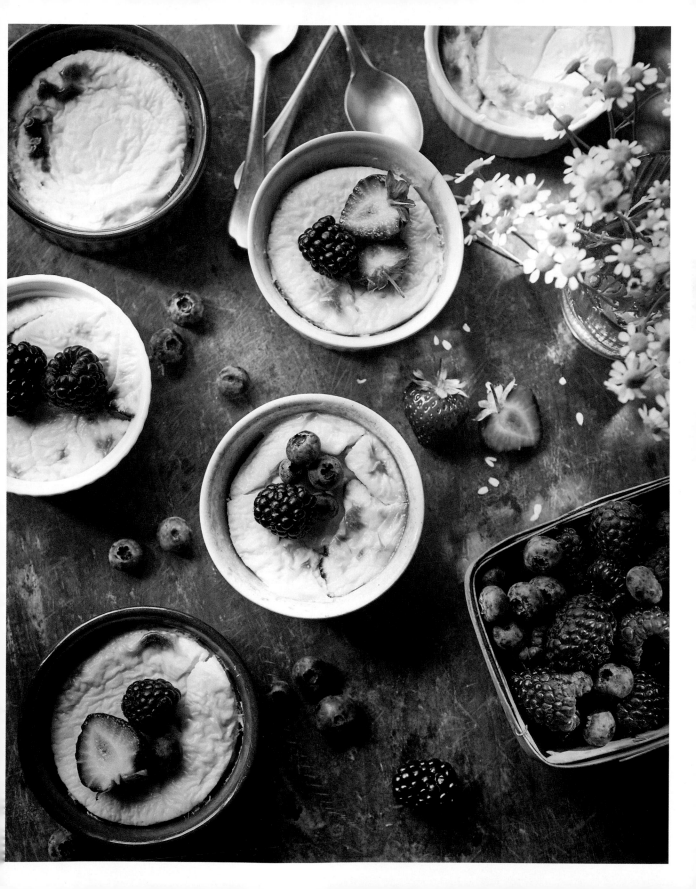

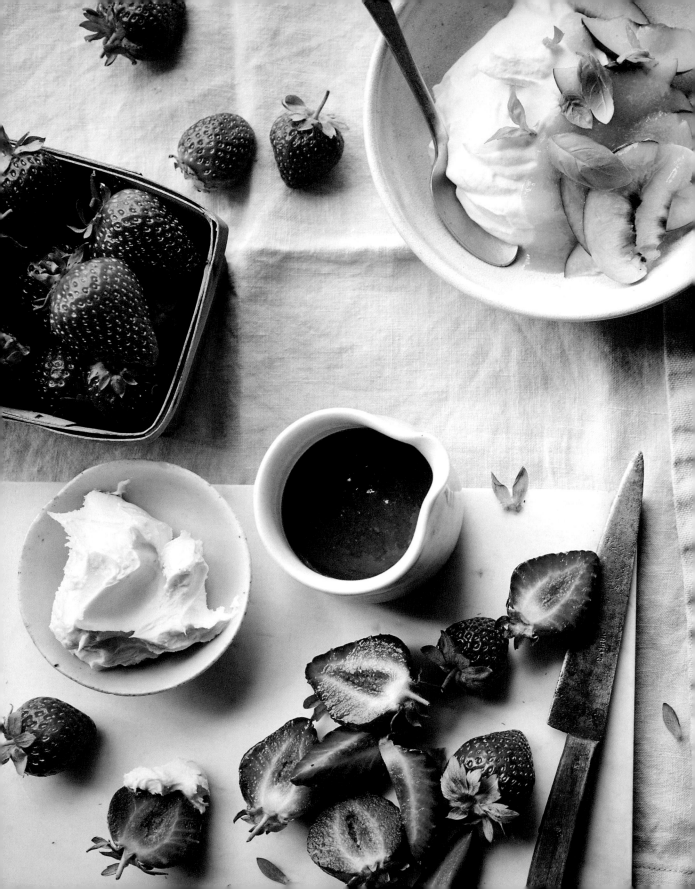

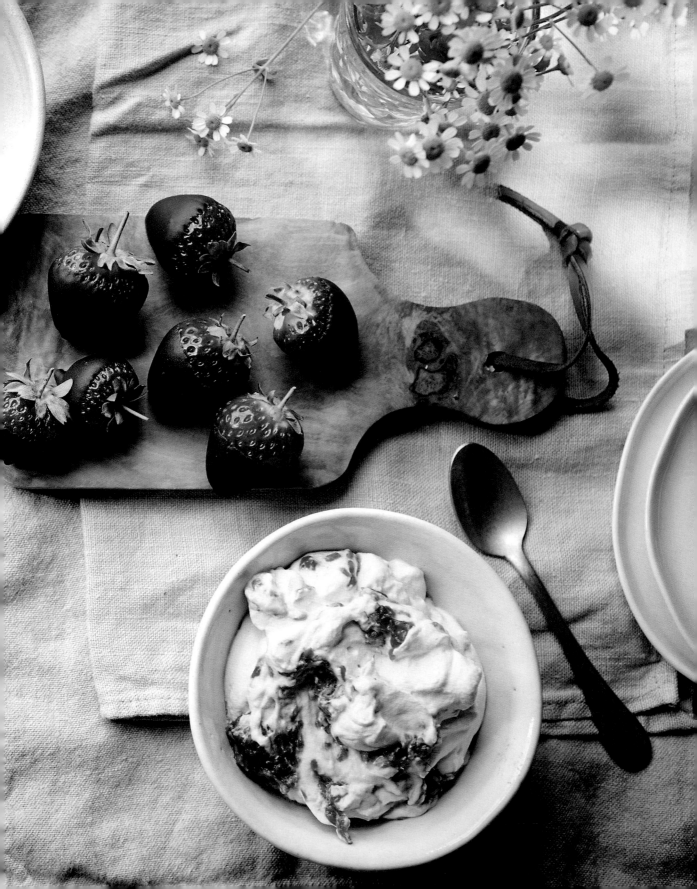

SUPER SIMPLE SPEEDY DESSERTS

These are recipes to whip up in a hurry. Apart from David's Heaven, all of these recipes serve 4.

David's Heaven

Dr David Unwin's idea of heaven is to share a bowl of fresh, large strawberries with his grandchildren. He halves them and they top each one with clotted cream. There's no hint of sugar and everyone is happy.

Per serving of 1 large strawberry (25g/1oz) plus 10g (¼oz) clotted cream 1.6g net carbs, 0.5g fibre, 0.3g protein, 6.5g fat, 66kcal

Nectarines, Basil & Cream

I have noticed in all my fruity experiments that if you crush or purée fruit, then you seem to get more flavour from it than if you leave it whole. If you don't have nectarines, use peaches or apricots instead or open and drain a can of similar fruit.

Cut 1 nectarine into quarters and purée it with 1 tablespoon of rum (optional) and 1 teaspoon of honey, if the fruit isn't sweet. Slice 3 nectarines and throw on to a serving plate. Pour over the purée and scatter over a handful of basil leaves. Whip 100ml (3½fl oz) double cream to soft peaks and serve with the fruit.

Per serving (with rum and honey) 14.7g net carbs, 2.4g fibre, 2g protein, 8.1g fat, 150kcal

Giancarlo's Gorgeous Raspberry Cream

The Unwins showed us this recipe a couple of years ago and Giancarlo has been making it ever since. Simply whisk 150ml (5fl oz) double cream, 2 teaspoons of vanilla extract, 1 teaspoon of honey (if the fruit isn't very sweet) and 250g (9oz) raspberries or strawberries together by hand or in a mixer with the whisk attachment. As it mixes, the berries will break down and mix with the cream, giving a beautifully light pink dessert.

Per serving 5.8g net carbs, 4g fibre, 1.3g protein, 19.3g fat, 219kcal

Fresh Berry Sauce

This is ideal to make with soft fruit slightly past its best. Use a fork or a stick blender to mash 250g (9oz) hulled strawberries or raspberries, blueberries or a mixture of berries. Stir in 1 teaspoon of vanilla extract and, if the fruit is very sour, 1 teaspoon of honey. If you like it, add 1 tablespoon of white rum. You should have a pulpy, thick jam that can be swirled into or poured over ricotta or whipped cream. My mother would often make a fresh raspberry sauce and pour it over fresh strawberries or the other way around.

Per serving (with rum) 4.2g net carbs, 1.2g fibre, 0.4g protein, 0.1g fat, 37kcal

Chocolate-coated Strawberries

Sweet, ripe strawberries with bitter, dark chocolate are always a hit. Put 400g (14oz) strawberries on to a small tray and chill in the freezer for 5 minutes. Melt 100g (3½oz) dark chocolate (at least 85% cocoa solids) in a heatproof bowl over a saucepan of simmering water without letting the bowl touch the water. Alternatively melt the chocolate in the microwave. Simply dip the very cold strawberries into the chocolate and then lay them on baking parchment back on the tray. Return to the fridge or freezer for a few minutes just to set and serve straight away or leave in the fridge for up to a day.

Per serving 10.5g net carbs, 6g fibre, 3.8g protein, 11.8g fat, 178kcal

Chocolate Fondants

SERVES 8

150g (5½oz) butter, softened, plus
  extra for greasing

150g (5½oz) dark chocolate (85%
  cocoa solids), broken into small pieces

2 Medjool dates, stoned and
  finely chopped

6 eggs

100g (3½oz) ground almonds

2 teaspoons vanilla extract

Per serving 9.4g net carbs, 4.7g fibre,
9.2g protein, 34g fat, 394kcal

This indulgent dessert is a luxury treat and although we've used two dates and sugar in the form of chocolate, this fondant has fewer carbs than traditional versions, which can contain up to 56g (2oz) carbs and 670 calories. If you are in a hurry, the desserts can be made in a food processor. Also, if you want to make them ahead of time to serve later, keep them chilled and allow 10 minutes to cook. Any leftover cooked fondants can be eaten the next day as deliciously gooey brownies.

Preheat the oven to 220°C/200°C fan/425°F/gas mark 7. Grease 8 x 5cm (2in) metal moulds or ramekins with butter. Line the base of each one with a small circle of baking parchment. A roughly torn circle will do.

Melt the chocolate in the microwave until just soft or put it into a heatproof bowl over a saucepan of barely simmering water, but not touching the water. Once the chocolate has melted, stir through and set aside.

Mash the chopped dates with 2 tablespoons of very hot water in a mixing bowl, using a fork to create a purée. Add the butter and beat together with an electric mixer or food processor until pale and fluffy.

Add 3 eggs, followed by half the almonds and the vanilla and whisk to combine. Then add the remaining eggs and almonds followed by the melted chocolate, whisking to combine.

Divide the mixture between the moulds or ramekins; they should not be more than two thirds full. Put them on a tray and cook for 8 minutes or until just firm to the touch.

Serve the fondants in the ramekins or gently turn out on to a plate to serve. Eat them straight away on their own, with raspberries, thick Greek yogurt or cream. Keep any leftover cooked fondants in the fridge for up to 3 days.

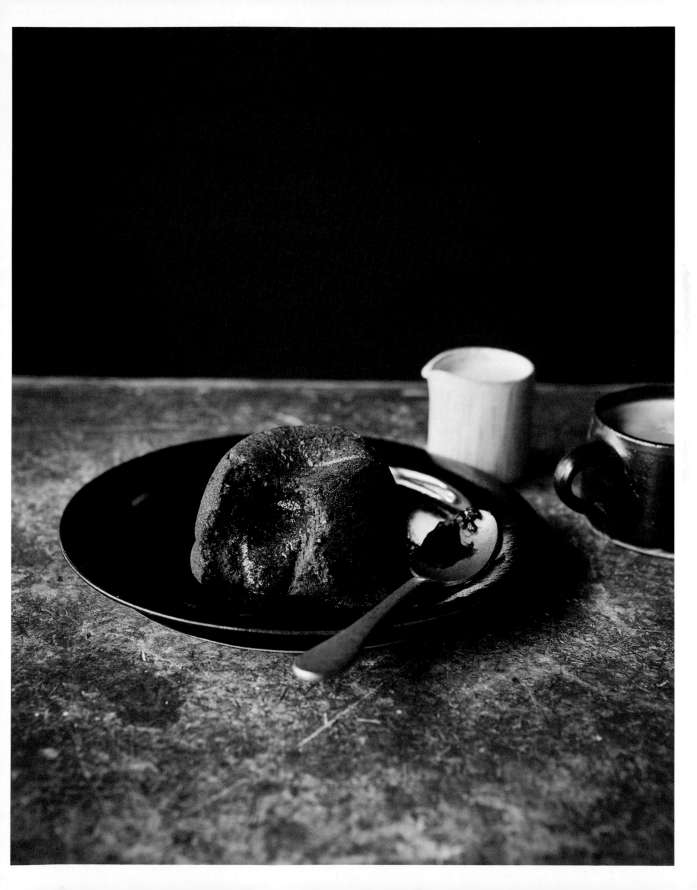

Baked Fruit & Coconut Custard

SERVES 6

750g (1lb 10z) plums, peaches, apricots, nectarines or apples, thinly sliced, and/or berries

6 teaspoons rum or another liqueur (optional)

1 tablespoon vanilla extract

zest and juice of 1 orange or ground cinnamon, to taste

For the coconut custard

10g (¼oz) cornflour

400g (14oz) can coconut milk

3 egg yolks

2 teaspoons vanilla extract

2 teaspoons honey

Per serving of baked fruit 14.3g net carbs, 1.7g fibre, 0.1g protein, 0.3g fat, 81kcal
Per serving of coconut custard 6.5g net carbs, 0.5g fibre, 2.4g protein, 14.2g fat, 161kcal

These parhcment parcels are a hit all year round. They are great for using overripe fruit as well as bringing out the flavour in hard fruit, as both are softened in the cooking process. Try combos like frozen berries and kirsch in spring, strawberry and peach in summer, apple and blackberry in autumn, and apple, orange and rum in winter. I like to do individual parcels to serve to guests in bowls so they can eat out of them but you can easily make fewer larger parcels if easier. Dry fruits such as apples benefit from a splash of water to help them cook. Serve on their own, with the Coconut Custard recipe below or whipped cream or thick Greek yogurt.

Preheat the oven to 220°C/200°C fan/425°F/gas mark 7. Cut 6 pieces of baking parchment into 36cm (14in) squares.

Lay 125g (4½oz) of the fruit in the centre of each piece of baking parchment and splash over 1 teaspoon of the rum, if using, ½ teaspoon of vanilla, a squeeze of orange juice and ¼ teaspoon of orange zest or a pinch of cinnamon.

Fold two opposite edges of the parchment up to meet each other above the fruit. Make a fold of both pieces together of about 2cm (¾in), then fold again. Do this several times until the fold is about 4cm (1½in) above the food. Now twist the ends like a sweet. Place the parcels on a baking tray to cook for 10–15 minutes depending on the ripeness of the fruit. You can feel when the fruit is soft by pressing lightly on the parcels.

Meanwhile, make the coconut custard. Put all the ingredients in a medium saucepan and whisk them together, while cold, until smooth. Now move the saucepan on to a medium–high heat and continue to whisk until it has thickened. Remove from the heat and decant into a jug. Use straight away or keep warm until serving. To stop a skin forming, cover the surface with a damp piece of baking parchment.

Remove the fruit parcels from the oven and carefully transfer them to soup or dessert dishes. Ask everyone to unwind the ends to reveal the fruit inside but be aware of the steam and hot juices. Serve with the coconut custard.

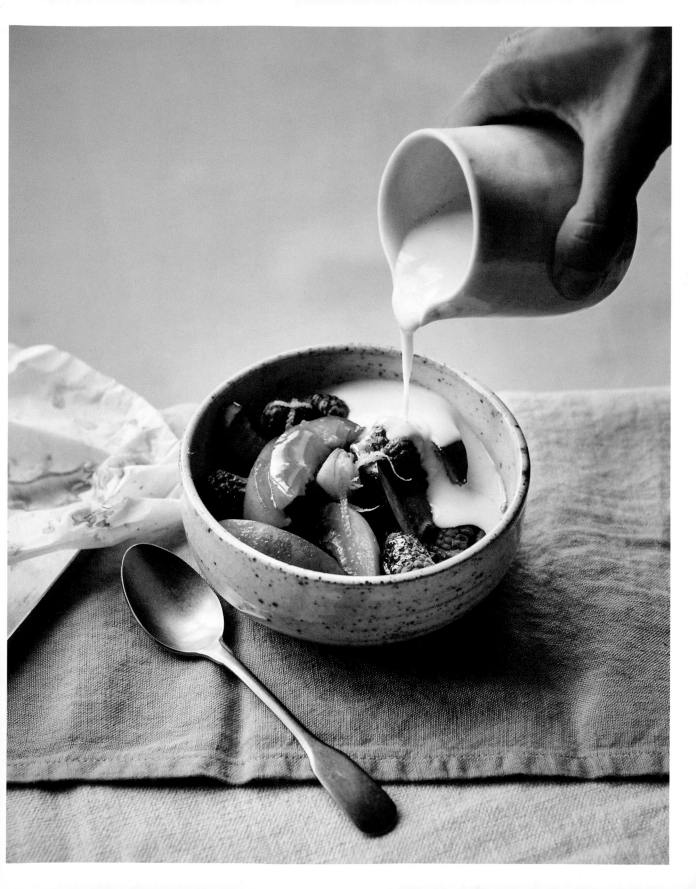

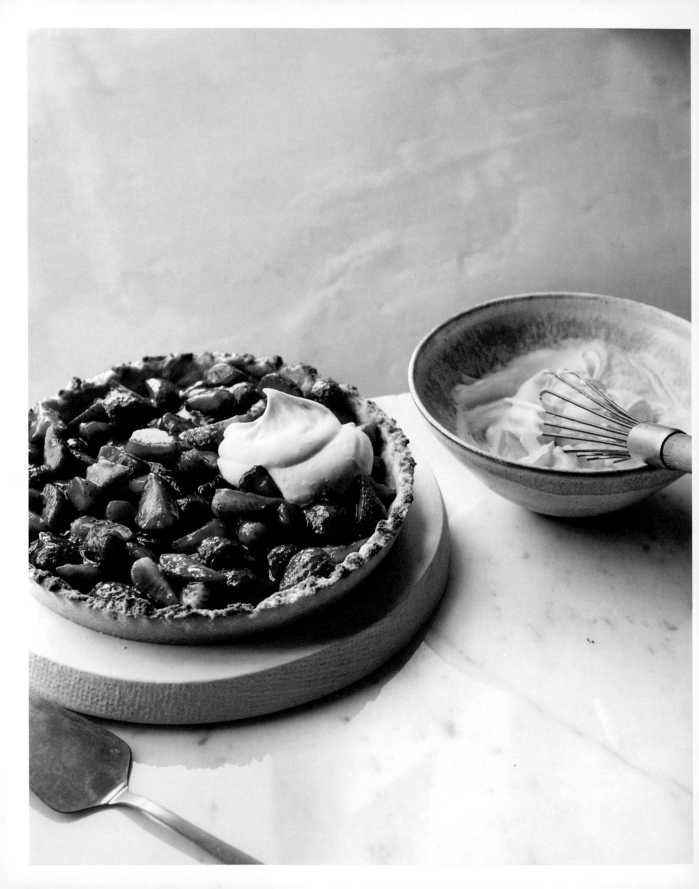

Strawberry & Cream Pie

SERVES 8

500g (1lb 2oz) strawberries

200ml (7fl oz) whipping cream

1 teaspoon vanilla extract

1 teaspoon honey

For the pastry

2 teaspoons honey

75g (2½oz) butter, softened and
    cut into small cubes

100g (3½oz) ground almonds

50g (1¾oz) coconut flour

finely grated zest of 1 small lemon or
    ½ orange (optional)

1 teaspoon vanilla extract

1 egg

Per serving 9g net carbs, 4.8g fibre,
5.1g protein, 28.1g fat, 322kcal

This stunning dessert is not off-limits even when living a low-carb lifestyle. Use any seasonal, ripe, low-carb fruit if strawberries aren't in season, such as apricots, plums, berries or apples that are naturally sweet, so you won't need any added sugar. The pastry is flavoured with lemon or orange zest, which is how the Italians make theirs, but it's not essential if you don't have any citrus fruit.

Preheat the oven to 220°C/200°C fan/425°F/gas mark 7. Line a 22cm (8½in) tart tin with a circle of baking parchment about 4cm (1½in) larger than the tin.

Mix all the pastry ingredients together in a bowl with a spoon or blitz briefly in a food processor until just combined; don't over-mix or the pastry will be too soft to use straight away. Press the pastry into the prepared tin. Use your hands to push the pastry to form a case about 1.5cm (⅝in) thick. Prick a few holes in the pastry base with a fork to stop it rising. Bake for 8–10 minutes or until firm to the touch and golden brown all over.

Remove the pastry from the oven and use the parchment to lift it carefully on to a cooling rack. After a couple of minutes, carefully slide the parchment out from the bottom so the pastry can cool quicker.

While the tart is cooling, hull the strawberries. Purée 150g (5½oz) of the strawberries and quarter the remaining fruit. Mix the purée with the sliced strawberries and set aside.

Whip the cream with the vanilla and honey until it forms soft peaks, then set aside in the fridge.

As soon as the pastry has almost cooled to room temperature, transfer it to a serving plate. You can use the base of a loose-bottomed cake tin to transfer it from tray to plate.

Pour the strawberry mixture over the pastry and top with the whipped cream. Serve straight away or chill for up to a day in the fridge.

Sicilian Ricotta Creams

SERVES 4

40g (1½oz) whole blanched almonds, pistachios, macadamia or walnuts

250g (9oz) ricotta

1 heaped teaspoon ground cinnamon

2 teaspoons honey

2 teaspoons vanilla extract

2 tablespoons dark rum (optional)

½ teaspoon finely grated satsuma, clementine or orange zest

15g (½oz) dark chocolate (85% cocoa solids), finely chopped

Per serving 9.4g net carbs, 1.8g fibre, 7.3g protein, 13g fat, 207kcal

I have spent many a day peering into Sicilian patisseries, fascinated by their use of local ricotta, fruit, almonds, pistachios and plenty of sugar. This dessert is based on *cuccia*, an old, little-known recipe made with wheatberries in sweet ricotta once a year for the Feast of Santa Lucia. It is unusual, but we love it; the cream is soft and perfumed with orange and cinnamon with the bonus crunch of nuts and chocolate. I like to serve it in espresso cups and use coffee spoons to eat it. The servings are not big, but they are filling, and are the perfect end to a dinner with friends.

Preheat the oven to 220°C/200°C fan/425°F/gas mark 7.

Spread the nuts out on a baking tray and cook for 6 minutes or until lightly browned. Tip on to a plate to cool to room temperature.

Whisk the ricotta with all the remaining ingredients, except the chocolate, in a small bowl. Mix 30g (1oz) of the cooled nuts and the chocolate into the cream then taste the mixture. Add more cinnamon or orange zest to your taste. Spoon into 4 small glasses or espresso cups and top with the remaining nuts. Any leftovers will keep for a couple of days in the fridge.

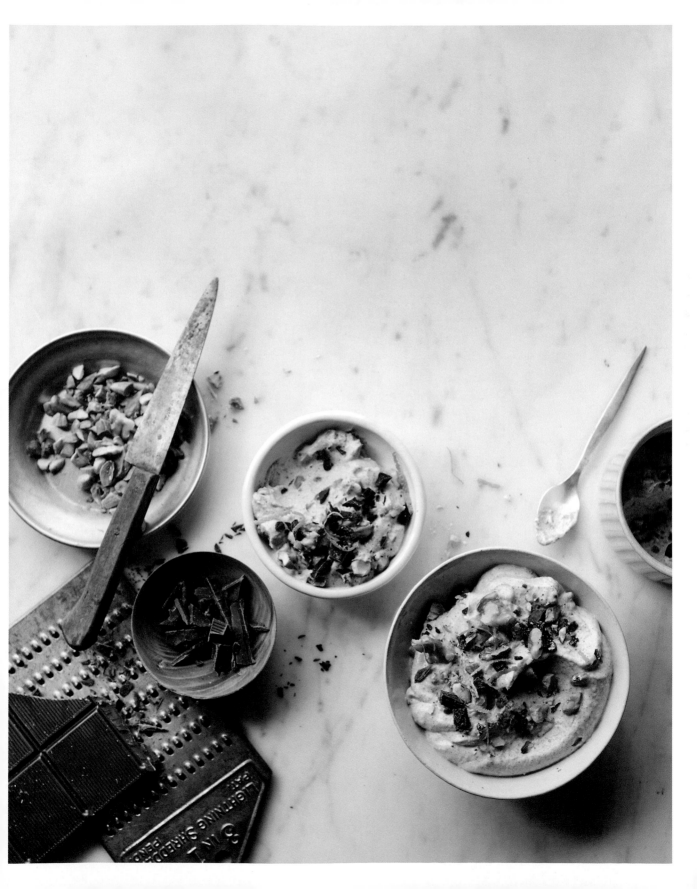

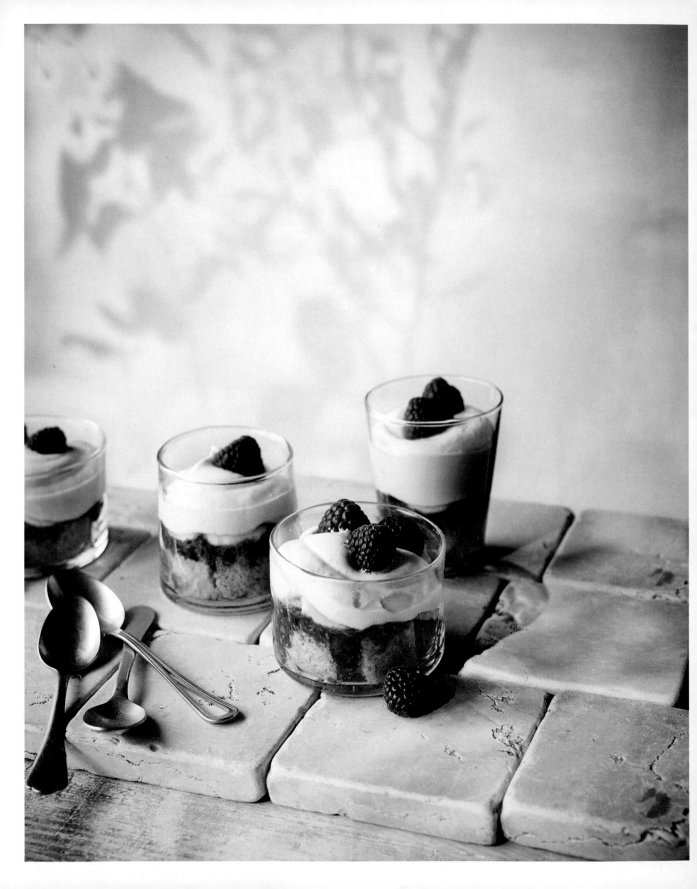

Sherry Trifle

SERVES 4

125g (4½oz) fresh or frozen
   raspberries, plus a handful
   to decorate

½ teaspoon vanilla extract

8 teaspoons dry sherry or dark rum

1 small banana, sliced

For the sponge

100g (3½oz) ground almonds

2 eggs

20g (¾oz) butter, softened

1 teaspoon baking powder

2 teaspoons vanilla extract

2 teaspoons honey

For the cream

100g (3½oz) mascarpone

1 egg, separated

1 teaspoon honey

1 tablespoon vanilla extract

75ml (2½fl oz) double cream

Per serving 16.8g net carbs, 5.4g
fibre, 11g protein, 42g fat, 534kcal

Ta-dah, trifle! I love to serve this as guests never expect me to indulge in rich puddings any more. However, with a few adaptations it's possible to enjoy treats such as this once in a while. If good fresh raspberries aren't available, use frozen raspberries to make the jam and use toasted almonds to decorate the trifles. To reduce the net carbs to just 10g (¼oz) a serving, omit the banana.

Beat the sponge ingredients together in a bowl until smooth, then transfer to a microwavable container, such as a heatproof shallow bowl or 2 mugs. The shape isn't important as you can cut the sponge to fit later. Microwave on full power for 1½–2 minutes or until firm to the touch. Alternatively cook the sponge in parchment-lined or silicone muffin moulds at 200°C/180°C fan/400°F/gas mark 6 for 12–15 minutes.

As soon as the sponge is cooked, tip it out and leave to cool for 5 minutes. When it is cool enough to handle, cut it into 1.5cm (⅝in) slices and set aside to cool to room temperature.

Mash the raspberries with the vanilla and set aside. Fresh raspberries might need an extra tablespoon of water as the juices need to soak into the sponge. If your raspberries were frozen and then defrosted, they will probably be juicy enough.

When the sponges have cooled to room temperature, divide them between 4 serving bowls or wide glasses. You can cut or tear them to fit. Pour 2 teaspoons of rum over each one and then spoon over the mashed raspberries. Divide the sliced banana between the bowls.

Whisk the mascarpone, egg yolk, honey and vanilla together with an electric mixer or hand whisk until well combined and creamy. Add the cream and whisk again until the mixture is firm.

Whisk the egg white to soft peaks with a clean and dry whisk and fold lightly into the cream mixture in two batches. Divide the cream between the bowls and top with the whole raspberries.

Syllabub

SERVES 6

100g (3½oz) mascarpone
300ml (10fl oz) double cream
1 tablespoon honey
100ml (3½fl oz) dry white wine

Per serving 4.9g net carbs, 0g fibre,
1.5g protein, 31.5g fat, 318kcal

This creamy, light and nostalgic dessert reminds me of my parents' 1970s dinner parties. I loved it then and it is great to recreate now, just minus the sugar.

Whisk the mascarpone, cream and honey together in a mixing bowl until firm. Add the wine a little at a time and keep whisking until it is combined. Divide between 6 glasses and serve straight away or chill for up to a day before eating. Any leftovers will keep for a day in the fridge.

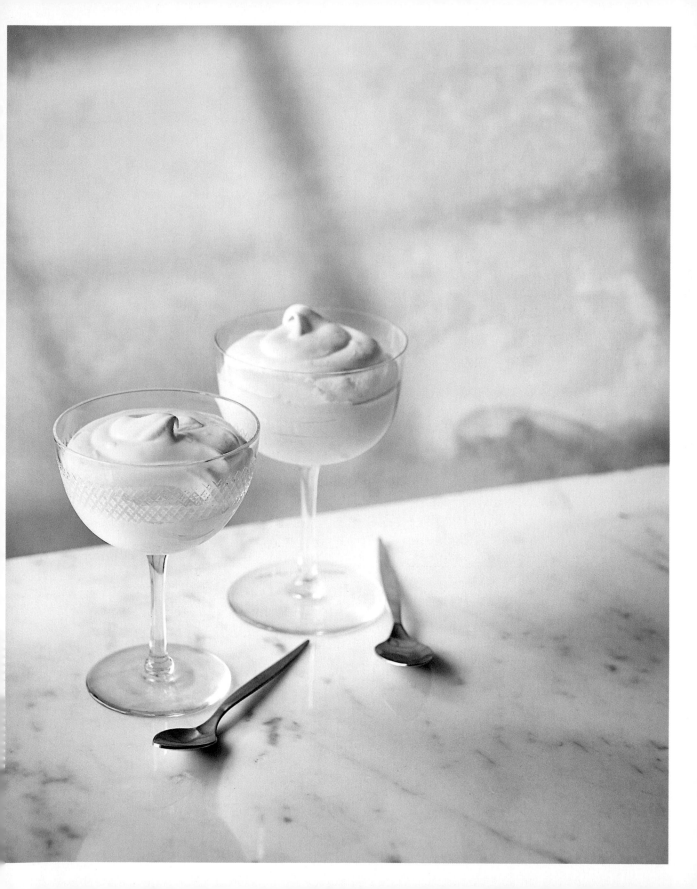

Peach Melba

SERVES 4

150g (5½oz) frozen or fresh raspberries, plus 12 to decorate

2 teaspoons vanilla extract

1 teaspoon honey (optional)

4 fresh or drained, canned peaches

200ml (7fl oz) whipping cream

Per serving 17.9g net carbs, 5.5g fibre, 3.4g protein, 18.6g fat, 266kcal

This wonderful dessert can be made with fresh peaches in summer or drained, canned peaches in winter. Cooking berries gives them a naturally sweet jammy taste; use up soft berries or frozen ones. Serve the sauce hot or cold on the peaches, or try it with yogurt, cream or whipped coconut cream.

Put the raspberries (you can do this from frozen) and 1 teaspoon of the vanilla in a saucepan. Bring to the boil and use a potato masher to mash them to a pulp as they cook and soften. Reduce the heat to low and simmer gently for 5 minutes, stirring frequently. You should be left with a sauce with a pouring, soup-like consistency. If it is very runny, heat the sauce for a further few minutes to reduce and thicken it. If the raspberries are sweet, don't add the honey. Pour the sauce into a cold, shallow bowl to cool quickly.

Slice the peaches and put into glasses or bowls to serve.

Whip the cream and remaining vanilla until the cream forms soft peaks. Spoon over the peaches. When the sauce has cooled to room temperature, pour it over the cream and serve straight away, decorated with the whole raspberries.

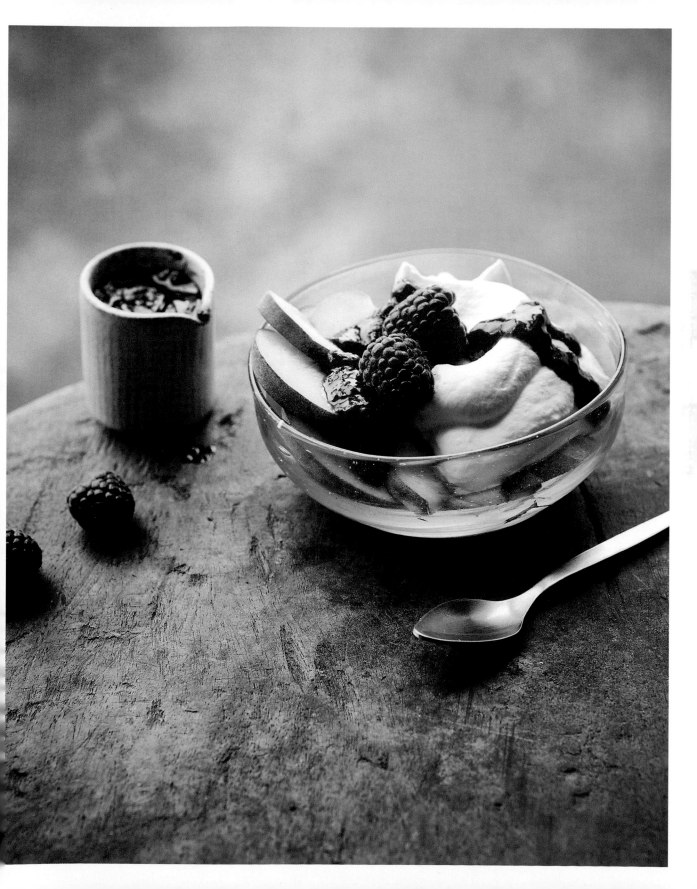

Cinnamon & Apple Yogurt

SERVES 2

1 medium apple

½ teaspoon ground cinnamon

2 teaspoons vanilla extract

300g (10½oz) Greek yogurt

50g (1¾oz) pecans or walnuts, roughly chopped

2 tablespoons sunflower or pumpkin seeds, plus extra to decorate

Per serving 21.3g net carbs, 5.8g fibre, 11.7g protein, 40g fat, 489kcal

This is delicious as a fast dessert or even for breakfast. Enjoy as it is or top with a few berries. If you want to be extra quick, don't cook the apples, just stir them in with the other ingredients and omit the water.

Chop the apple into pieces no bigger than 1cm (½in); there is no need to peel it but do discard the core.

Put the apple into a small frying pan or saucepan with the cinnamon, 1 teaspoon of the vanilla and 2 tablespoons of water. Cover with a lid and bring to the boil. Bubble for 2 minutes over a high heat, shaking the pan occasionally. Remove the lid and cook for a further 2 minutes to evaporate the water. Tip the apple on to a plate and spread it out to cool.

Meanwhile, mix the yogurt with the remaining vanilla, nuts and seeds. When the apple has cooled to room temperature, mix it with the yogurt and serve in glasses with some seeds on top. Eat straight away or chill until you are ready. They will last in the fridge for a couple of days.

Raspberry & Lemon Cookies

MAKES 20 (4CM/1½IN) COOKIES

225g (8oz) ground almonds

*25g (1oz) butter, softened, plus extra
    for greasing*

½ teaspoon baking powder

1 egg white

2 teaspoons honey

2 teaspoons vanilla extract

finely grated zest of ½ lemon

75g (2½oz) raspberries

Per cookie 1.9g net carbs, 1.3g fibre,
2.5g protein, 7g fat, 84kcal

Eat these cookies as they are or crumble them over yogurt, cream or fruit. They become soft after a day but can easily be re-baked in a hot oven for a couple of minutes to firm up. Save the egg yolk for an omelette or scrambled eggs. If you have leftover raspberries, push one into the top of each cookie before you bake them.

Preheat the oven to 200°C/180°C fan/400°F/gas mark 6 and grease a baking tray.

Put all the ingredients in a bowl and use a metal spoon to stir them together, breaking up the raspberries as you go.

Use a teaspoon to pick up a walnut-sized ball of the mixture. Use another teaspoon to scrape the ball off and drop it on the prepared tray. Repeat the process until you have about 20 rough mounds of cookie mixture on the tray. They keep their shape as they cook but leave at least a two-finger-width gap between them.

Bake for 10 minutes or until golden brown and firm to the touch. Leave to cool for 5 minutes before transferring the cookies to a wire rack. When they have cooled to room temperature, the cookies can be stored in an airtight container for 2 days or for 5 days in the fridge. If they become soft, re-bake them at 180°C/160°C fan/350°F/gas mark 4 for 3–5 minutes to firm up.

Mini Banana Muffins

MAKES 12 MINI MUFFINS

2 ripe bananas, weighing about
    130g (4½oz) each

100g (3½oz) walnuts

75g (2½oz) carrot, scrubbed

100g (3½oz) ground almonds

50g (1¾oz) butter, softened,
    plus extra for greasing (optional)

2 eggs

1 heaped teaspoon baking powder

For the topping

2 teaspoons honey

180g (6oz) cream cheese

1 tablespoon vanilla extract

Per muffin 8.4g net carbs, 2.2g fibre,
5.3g protein, 18.6g fat, 212kcal

It might seem incongruous to include a low-carb banana treat, especially when we have told you how many teaspoons of sugar one banana is equivalent to (see page 11), but the natural sweetness of the fruit is shared between 12 servings here, so the banana muffin can be back on the menu. We have omitted flour and sugar and used wholesome nuts, seeds and carrot instead.

Preheat the oven to 220°C/200°C fan/425°F/gas mark 7. Use a silicone mini muffin mould or grease a metal mini muffin tin.

Mash the bananas in a mixing bowl with a fork and set aside.

Blitz the walnuts in a food processor until you have a combination of textures between small gravel and sand. Tip them into the bowl with the banana.

Coarsely grate the carrot in a food processor or by hand and add to the bowl with the remaining cake ingredients. Stir together until well combined.

Pour this mixture into the muffin tin and bake for 12–15 minutes or a skewer comes out clean when inserted into the centre of the muffins. Leave to cool in the tin for 3 minutes before transferring to a wire rack.

Make the topping by mixing all the ingredients together. Serve on the side of the warm muffins. Enjoy straight away or leave to cool to room temperature, then chill in the fridge. The muffins will keep, chilled, for up to 3 days.

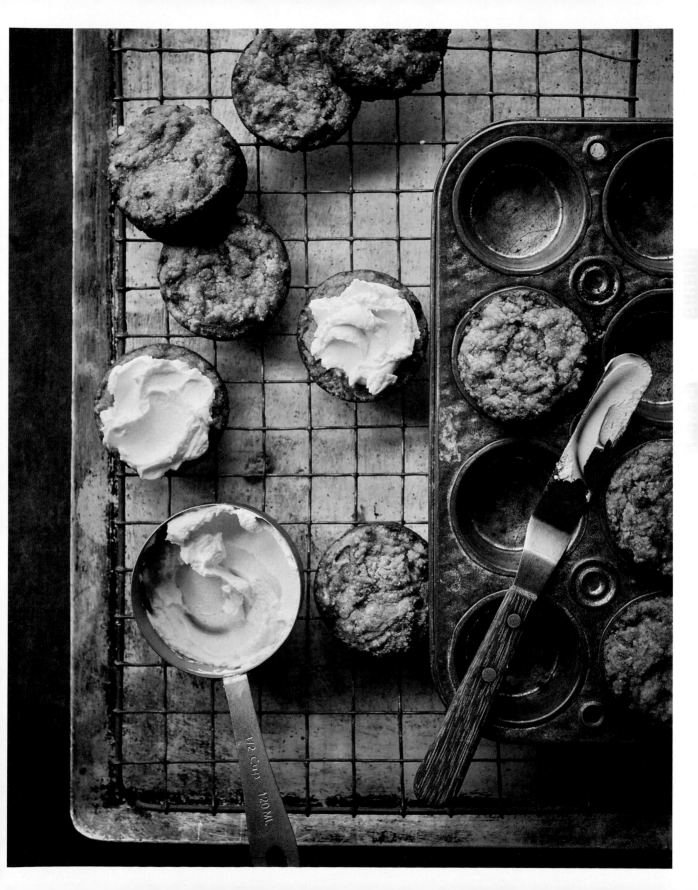

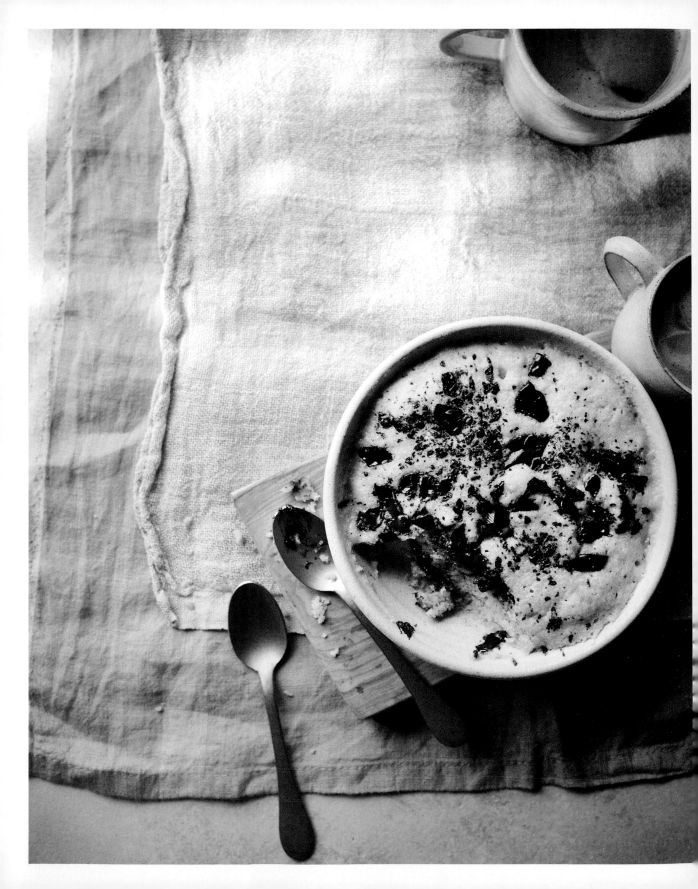

Instant Chocolate & Tahini Indulgence

SERVES 2

50g (1¾oz) grounds almonds

1 egg

1 teaspoon vanilla extract

1 heaped tablespoon tahini or crunchy peanut butter

2 tablespoons double cream

1 teaspoon honey

½ teaspoon baking powder

12g (½oz) dark chocolate (85% cocoa solids), finely chopped

Per serving 8.1g net carbs, 4.1g fibre, 10g protein, 29.6g fat, 350kcal

This very quick cake is miraculously speedy and totally delicious. Microwave in the dish and eat from that for a dessert in a hurry. If you prefer to cook the cake in the oven, it takes about 8 minutes at 200°C/180°C fan/400°F/gas mark 6. Enjoy the cake on its own or indulge further with double cream.

Mix all the ingredients, apart from the chocolate, together in a bowl (if the tahini is very stiff add a spoonful of hot water first to loosen it) and pour into a small microwavable dish to share or divide between 2 microwavable teacups. Scatter over the chocolate and microwave on full power for 1½–2 minutes or until firm to the touch.

Leave to cool for 5 minutes before eating.

Flaxseed Oatcakes

SERVES 6/MAKES 36 BISCUITS

75g (2½oz) rolled oats

75g (2½oz) ground golden flaxseed (linseed)

¼ teaspoon bicarbonate of soda

30g (1oz) butter

scant 1 teaspoon salt

Per 30g serving 7.4g net carbs, 4.6g fibre, 4g protein, 10.1g fat, 150kcal

I was tempted to suggest that this was a rare Scottish recipe from the Highlands, but in fact it is simply my way to reduce the carbs in traditional oatcakes by substituting flaxseed (also known as linseed) for oats. These are ideal slathered in butter while still warm, topped with cheese or prettied up with cream cheese, smoked salmon and dill for an occasion. They can be flavoured with chopped rosemary, black onion (nigella) seeds or a whole host of other flavours. They are also good for lunchboxes. If you can find golden flaxseed, the colour will be more golden than the darker variety but both do the job.

Cut two pieces of baking parchment the size of your largest oven tray and set aside.

Use a food processor (not a small one or the mixture will stick to the sides) to grind the oats into a flour. Add the remaining ingredients plus 3 tablespoons of water and whizz together for a few seconds until the mixture is well combined. If the mixture is very dry, add another teaspoon of water and whizz again.

Preheat the oven to 220°C/200°C fan/425°F/gas mark 7.

Put one piece of baking parchment on to the work surface and transfer the dough on to it. Put the other piece of baking parchment over the top and roll out the pastry into a rough rectangle. Peel off the top sheet and neaten the rectangle by cutting it with a cook's knife and patchworking pieces of the dough off and adding them in as necessary. The rectangle should be 5mm (¼in) thick. Slide the parchment with the dough on to the oven tray.

Now shape the oatcakes by cutting 5 lines across and 5 lines down with a cook's knife to divide the dough into 36 smaller rectangles/squares. Alternatively, you can leave the dough whole and break it into shards of oatcakes after cooking. Bake for 10–12 minutes, then leave to cool to room temperature.

Serve straight away or store in an airtight container for up to 5 days.

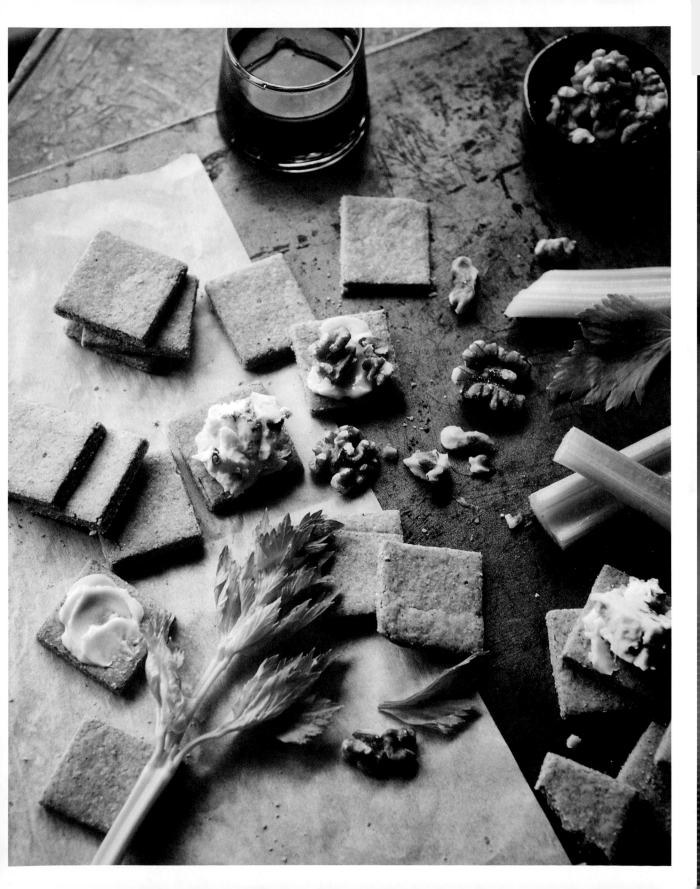

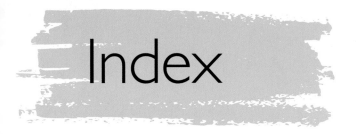

Index

RESOURCES & REFERENCES

The nutritional analysis was mainly calculated using **Cronometer** software. However, I would point out that calculating carbs, fibre, protein, fat and calories doesn't seem an exact science. When cross-checking analysis from other sources there were discrepancies between all of them, sometimes large. I felt Cronometer lay roughly in the middle so used this as my preferred software on these recipes. Know what you are eating and don't worry too much about counting things – that is my message.

Carbs and Cals is a useful app and book to have if only to familiarize yourself with carb values.

FreeStyle Libre makes instant glucose monitoring systems and can be found at **www.freestylelibre.co.uk**

The Public Health Collaboration is a charity dedicated to informing and implementing decisions for better public health. Find out more at **www.phcuk.org**

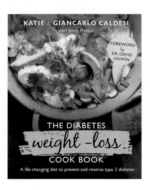
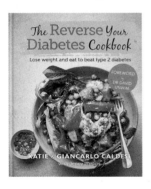

SOCIAL MEDIA

To follow Katie and Giancarlo Caldesi on social media please see **@katiecaldesi** on Instagram and Twitter and our Facebook pages **LowCarbTogether** and **Caldesi Italian Restaurants**.

For information about our restaurants see **www.caldesi.com**

For information on cookery courses at our schools or online see **www.lowcarbtogether.com** and **www.caldesi.com**

Follow Dr David Unwin on Twitter **@lowcarbGP**

Dr Jen Unwin is on Twitter as **@jen_unwin**

Find Jenny Phillips on Twitter **@JennyNutrition** and **www.inspirednutrition.co.uk**

Our LOW CARB TOGETHER Website

www.lowcarbtogether.com is our website packed full of up-to-date information and resources to help you on your low-carb journey.

Along with new recipes and links to developments in the low-carb community, discover other medical conditions helped by a low-carb lifestyle, baking tips, nut-free, egg-free and gluten-free recipes, useful suppliers, cooking videos and much more.

You'll also find details of low-carb events, online cookery courses and lots more besides.

ACKNOWLEDGEMENTS

A huge thank you to:

Everyone who suggested and tested recipes with me for this book including Anne Hudson, Jenny Phillips, Stefano Borella, Carly Roberts, the Skatcho family, the Soin family and more.

And to the patient friends and family who read the proofs and gave their opinions and corrections including: Charlotte Soin, Brian McLeod, Lou and Phil Ford and Philip Beresford.

Vicky Orchard, editor.
Emily Noto, production.
Tina Smith Hobson for the book design.
Our agent, Jonathan Hayden.

The book is beautiful thanks to Maja Smend's stunning photography, Amy Stephenson's food styling and Nicole Theodorou's perfectly chosen props.

Giancarlo, Jenny and I were delighted to work with Dr David Unwin and Dr Jen Unwin on this project. Their knowledge, experience and help were invaluable. We wish it to be known that they have received no fee for their participation in this book. Instead we made a donation to the Public Health Collaboration to further their work spreading the real food message.